Praise for *Stumbling Toward Heaven*

"Mike Hamel nobly dealt with lymphoma that rapidly recurred and required a stem cell transplant to attain a remission. As he was recovering he was in a serious auto accident. He has persevered through difficulties that would destroy the faith of most people and is now even more thoughtful and gracious. We can all learn from his incredible struggles and triumphs."
 —Dr. Mark Brunvand, Hematologist/Oncologist

"My life's work involves shepherding heroic men and women through their cancer journeys. Every once in a while I find myself transformed by those I work with. Mike Hamel has been such a figure. Diagnosed with cancer in the prime of life, he has had to wrestle with his own faith while his body labored under the duress of chemotherapy. Mike offers us remarkable insights into the human condition and the capacity of the human spirit to triumph in the face of incredible adversity."
 —Dr. Dax Kurbegov, Oncologist

"Mike Hamel has written a deeply personal and courageous book, a raw and honest journal of his struggles, and of the challenge of survival and maintaining faith in the face of great adversity. *Stumbling Toward Heaven* is an invitation to experience the power of belief and the resilience of the human spirit. It's been a joy getting to know this remarkable author who is not 'slouching toward Bethlehem,' but stumbling forward mightily with grace and eloquence."
 —Lee Cantelon, author of *The Words*

"Fighting cancer has challenged Mike's fertile brain and struggling spirit as much as his fragile body and the story often seems more a conversation than a book. As reader and author walk together, none of us know where the road will lead, but even through our stumbling, both the journey and the destination become more real."
 —Dr. Carl Armerding, Professor and Former President of Regent College, Vancouver, B.C.

"The 'C' word typically evokes 'F' words —Fear, Flight, Fate, Freak, or Failure—from sufferers, families and friends alike. In *Stumbling Toward Heaven*, Mike Hamel rises above it all with an incredibly useful and unique approach; he's funny—and I mean really funny. Mike is a fabulous storyteller, capturing the essence of how one of life's many tragic realities cause us to re-examine the frailties of our faith. You don't have to be afflicted or affected by cancer to derive practical benefits from this book. The occurrence of the unexpected is an experience we all share in this life. It takes a gifted writer like Mike Hamel to help us make sense of it all and have some laughs along the way. Prescription: Buy This Book!"

—**Bill Dahl, Author, Creator of The Porpoise Diving Life (.com)**

"Have you ever reached a point when life got so hard that God seemed to disappear? St. John of the Cross called it the 'dark night of the soul.' Only it doesn't usually last a night. It can last for weeks, months, even years. When it's over, we rediscover the good news that God isn't disillusioned with us. He never had any illusions to begin with. I applaud my good friend Mike Hamel for telling his story as is, in motion, with honesty and humor. I only wish more of us could do the same."

—**David Sanford, author of *If God Disappears***

"*Stumbling Toward Heaven* is a personal meditation on what occurs when cancer besets a man and, through that man, an entire family. It is not about death, but about how the prospect of death concentrates the mind on those things that make life—even life with cancer—not just bearable but meaningful. Those who found insight in Randy Pausch's *The Last Lecture* will discover the same spirit here."

—**Jeff Rowes, Senior Attorney, Institute for Justice**

STUMBLING TOWARD HEAVEN

MIKE HAMEL

MY CANCER JOURNEY

Books by Mike Hamel

We Will Be Landing Shortly: Now What?
Lizzy the Leatherback
Giving Back
Executive Influence
The Entrepreneur's Creed

Matterhorn the Brave series:
   The Sword and the Flute
   Talis Hunters
   Pyramid Scheme
   Jewel Heist
   Dragon's Tale
   Rylan the Renegade
   Tunguska Event
   The Book of Stories
www.MatterhornTheBrave.com

TLC series:
   UFO on the Rez
   Bezer's Billions
   The Long Walk Home
   Zack's Cavern
www.TLCstories.com

Stumbling Toward Heaven

MIKE HAMEL
My Cancer Journey

To Susan:
My source of strength and claim to fame—
in this life and the next.
I want to be buried in a T-shirt that says,
I'M WITH HER!

CONTENTS

Preface   1

PART I—CANCER AND CHEMO   6
JUNE 2008 – FEBRUARY 2009

*Good News, It's Cancer!, Diffuse Large B-cell, Cancer 101,
In the Clinic, A Client Not a Patient, Farts and Fallout,
Flat as a Shadow, Blessed, Better Living through Drugs, Sleep on It,
Recovering Lymphomaniac*

PART II—RELAPSE AND TRANSPLANT   51
MARCH – AUGUST 2009

*Trouble in the Region, Transplant Prep, Reflections on Being Terminal,
In Hospital, Drugged Out, Read This Eat That, RMBMT-07-C,
Apheresis to Infusion, Aftermath, Home Again, Not Dead at 56*

PART III—ACCIDENT AND SURGERIES   101
AUGUST 2009 – DECEMBER 2010

*Tough Break, Getting Physical, Pain Scale, Typical Weeks,
What Are the Odds?, Pain and Purpose, Off the Cuff,
Size Doesn't Matter Much, Involuntary Recidivism, Candid Camera,
Temporary Condition, System Reboot, Road to Recovery,
Tale of Two Mikes*

PART IV —THE LONG SHADOW   159
JANUARY 2011 – AUGUST 2013

*Rituxan Regime, New Cancer, Neck Dissection, Recliner Reflections,
Shot in the Face, Noun and Verb, Drinking Downriver, Convalescence,
Unhappy Thanksgiving, Sneak Attack, Meditate on This,
Habits Old and New, The Hamel Diet, Symptom Free Not Pain Free,
Valentine's Day, Faustian Bargain*

Epilogue   229

PREFACE

Cancer is the leading cause of death worldwide, causing thirteen percent of all deaths on the planet: 7.6 million annually. About twenty-eight million people today have cancer, according to Dr. David Servan-Schreiber, himself a cancer patient. I joined their ranks in June 2008. For fifty-five years before that I had enjoyed robust health. Since then I have been cage-fighting with what Dr. Siddhartha Mukherjee calls the Emperor of all Maladies; each of us trying to get the other to tap out. (At 160 pounds I may be in the wrong sport, but, hey, I'm feisty.) This is a grudge match to the death that I aim to make last as long as possible.

I've had three bouts with cancer and the subsequent treatment has included a bone marrow transplant, thirty-six rounds of chemotherapy, thirty-three rounds of radiation and five surgeries. Ten weeks after my transplant, I was in a serious auto accident that resulted in a broken back, cracked sternum and ribs and a torn rotator cuff. (I've had three rotator cuff surgeries since then.) Due to a compromised immune system I've also contracted pneumonia several times and have lived with various other maladies.

I wrote this book to provide practical, firsthand information to those affected by cancer and other physical challenges. I took my computer and camera into offices, clinics, hospitals and ERs.

I interviewed doctors and nurses; I researched procedures and medications; I documented everything on my blog, OPEN Mike. Although it chronicles a life-and-death struggle, I've kept the tone casual, even humorous at times. It's part of how I cope. I choose to approach life in an upbeat manner, focusing on the positive and trying to learn from every experience. It was Mark Twain who said, "Humor is tragedy plus time."

The first version of this book (2011) included my physical problems and spiritual questions. I narrated three years of struggle as I lived them—unfiltered. But now I see the wisdom of separating the strands since most people with a deadly disease want useful information, not unsettling speculations. I also have two more years of adversity to chronicle, including the hardest blow of all, the sudden death of my wife, Susan. For these reasons I've revised *Stumbling* to focus on my physical trials and collected my spiritual musings in another book, *We Will Be Landing Shortly: Now What?*

These two books tell my story in my words. I hope they will help you better understand and tell yours.

o   o   o

"Anything that is not autobiography is plagiarism."
—Pedro Almodovar

PART I
CANCER AND CHEMO
JUNE 2008 – FEBRUARY 2009

"I'm going to beat this cancer or die trying."
—Michael Landon

GOOD NEWS, IT'S CANCER!

"I have good news," Dr. Dillon said, leaning forward on his elbows. "You have cancer. The biopsy shows the lump in your abdomen is non-Hodgkin lymphoma and not an omental tumor as the initial scan suggested."

Lymphoma is good news indeed. The first time I saw the good doctor a few weeks earlier he'd said, "You have a nonspecific mass in your omentum."

"I didn't even know I had an omentum," I replied.

"It's a fatty covering in the abdomen."

"How big is the mass?" ("Mass" sounds more benign than "tumor.")

"About the diameter of a grapefruit," he said, making a circle with thumbs and forefingers. "The nearby lymph nodes are also enlarged."

Dr. Dillon had no idea how long the tumor had been growing. I got introduced to it in the spring of 2008. I was getting low-grade cramps after sitting at my computer all day, which I put down to poor posture. Then I woke up two nights in a row with abdominal pain I couldn't blame on posture or indigestion. That's when I first felt the hardness in my gut.

The cramps went away about the time I made an appointment

with my family physician but the lump remained. I remember kneading my gut on the way to the doctor's trying to rekindle the pain that had caused me to make the appointment in the first place. Turns out I didn't have to worry about wasting the doctor's time; he could feel the abnormality and wouldn't buy my glib explanation that it was my abs of steel.

"It's only hard on one side," he pointed out.

"Okay," I conceded, "How about 'ab of steel'?"

"How about you get a CT scan?" he countered.

The scan revealed a mass large enough to warrant an immediate trip to a surgeon/oncologist, which is how I wound up at Dr. Dillon's.

Larry Dillon is a personable man with salt-and-pepper hair, an open face and straightforward manner. During our first visit he had explained to my wife, Susan, and me that the normal course of treatment is a complete surgical resection of the omentum. Before we left he warned about doing research on the Internet because the information on solid omental tumors "will scare you silly."

He got that right.

I had no problem finding authoritative articles on omental masses. I had hoped it was something Catholics attended during Lent, but no such luck. An article on eMedicine clinically stated, "Patients with primary malignant tumors of the omentum have a median survival time of only six months. Only 10-20% of patients are alive two years after surgical excision."

The word that popped out at me was "survival," a stark concept for a fifty-six-year-old who had seldom been sick and who had only been in a hospital as a visitor. Until then my closest brushes with mortality had been conducting funerals as a pastor. All that was about to change.

Since then I've been in and out of hospitals, clinics and doctor's offices. I have gone from a high-energy to a high-maintenance lifestyle, from avoiding even aspirin to popping up to twenty pills a day and having lethal doses of toxic chemicals injected directly into my chest.

Scan This, Biopsy That

The transition from diagnosis (determining what's wrong with a person), to prognosis (discerning how a disease will progress), is facilitated by a plethora of tests. The first was a CT scan, also called a CAT scan: Computed Axial Tomography. The results sent me to Dr. Dillon, who in turn ordered a biopsy of the mass in my abdomen.

The CT scan was invented in 1972 by a British engineer and a South African physicist, both of whom later received Nobel Prizes for their contributions to medicine and science. *Tomos* is Greek for "slice" and *graphia* means "without a knife." The CT scan uses X-rays and computers to examine the body in 3-D, which sure beats exploratory surgery! It allows radiologists to see abnormalities that, in the past, could only be found by surgeons—or coroners. Thankfully, the procedure is painless, unless you count drinking the contrast solution, which tastes like banana-flavored chalk.

I reported to Memorial Hospital on June 26 for my tumor biopsy. I remember talking to a nurse named Tammy while on the examination table and the next thing I knew I was in the recovery room an hour later. Thanks to the wonders of modern medicine and the skills of top-flight professionals, I can truly say the process was painless.

As I looked at my stomach after the biopsy, I noticed the "x" they made before the procedure was an inch below the actual cut. I pointed this out to Tammy, who explained that they'd marked me while I was holding my breath during the scan. Once I was under, I relaxed, hence the change in location.

The next day all I had to show for the biopsy was a small bruise and a slight soreness. I felt pretty upbeat but I was careful not to get too exuberant or else I'd pay the price. To an extent, I believe

Newton's Third Law also applies to emotions: "For every feeling, there is an equal and opposite feeling." Like other natural forces, emotions come finely balanced on a shifting fulcrum.

The hardest part of this ordeal so far had been telling family and friends and hearing the concern and tears in their voices. The possibility of a shortened life hadn't registered on me yet. I wasn't trying to suppress my feelings; they just hadn't gotten too worked up.

Obviously God had entered my thoughts but this crisis didn't suddenly cure my inability to pray. For a few years I'd suffered from the loss of a sense of God's presence. I'd been adrift in a spiritual Sargasso Sea, which may have contributed to my getting sick.

o   o   o

"Cancer is a word, not a sentence."
—John Diamond

DIFFUSE LARGE B-CELL

URING MY NEXT APPOINTMENT with Dr. Dillon, he gives me a copy of my biopsy report. The final diagnosis reads:

Diffuse Large B-cell Lymphoma
C2DO-Positive and BCL-2 Positive
Staining Pattern suggestive of Kappa Light Chain Restriction

In layman's terms, diffuse large B-cell lymphoma (DLBCL) is a common type of non-Hodgkin lymphoma (NHL), accounting for about two-in-five lymphomas. It's a cancer of the B-lymphocytes. Diffuse B-cell lymphoma can occur at any time between adolescence and old age and is slightly more common in men than women.

For practical purposes, non-Hodgkin lymphomas are also divided into one of two groups: low- and high-grade. Low-grade lymphomas are usually slow-growing, and high-grade lymphomas tend to grow more quickly. Diffuse large B-cell lymphoma is a high-grade lymphoma and needs prompt treatment. Chemotherapy is the use of anti-cancer (cytotoxic) drugs to destroy cancer cells. It is the main treatment for diffuse large B-cell lymphoma. The type of chemotherapy depends on the extent of the lymphoma and other factors, such as your age and general health (http://www.cancerbackup.org.uk/Cancertype/ Lymphomanon-Hodgkin/TypesofNHL/diffuselargeb-cell).

Lymphoma survivability (there's that word again) ranges from twenty-three percent to seventy-eight percent, depending on various factors. I'll get an idea of where I am on the continuum after more tests. I'm under sixty, in good physical shape and have no other conditions like high blood pressure or diabetes, all of which are in my favor.

I can't eat much without getting cramps due to the tumor crowding the rightful occupants of my abdomen. I can put splayed fingers on my gut and feel swelling at all four points of the handmade compass. Sort of like palming a softball. I've lost about ten pounds the last few months, which puts me at 5'10" and 160 pounds. Still, I feel fine and have no lack of energy. In Ashleigh Brilliant's slick little book, *I Have Abandoned My Search for Truth, And Am Now Looking for a Good Fantasy*, he notes that, "Inside every older person is a younger person wondering what happened." I could also say that, "Inside every sick person is a healthy person wondering what happened."

Testing Trifecta
Since lymphoma is a blood cancer, Dr. Dillon refers me to a hematologist/oncologist by the name of Dax Kurbegov. "Dax Kurbegov" sounds like a Russian spymaster but he's an American-born MD. I get a call from Dr. Kurbegov himself a few mornings later. He has no space in his schedule to see me until August. In the mean time I'll need to get a PET/CT scan, a bone marrow biopsy and a MUGA heart scan. These are in addition to the CT scan and tumor biopsy done earlier. I have no health insurance and these procedures cost a pretty penny. Oh well, better in debt

than dead I suppose.

The next day, July 9, I go in at 6:30 a.m. for the PET/CT that's used to diagnose and monitor treatment of certain cancers. A tracer element is injected into the body, usually fluorine-18 (fluorodeoxyglucose) that's taken up by glucose-using cells. Its concentration will reveal any rapidly growing malignancies.

PET/CT fusion imaging is most valuable for lung cancer and cancers located in regions of the body that have a complicated anatomy, such as the neck and lower pelvis. These areas of the body contain organs, tissue, muscles, bones, lymph nodes, air, fluids, etc., all in close proximity—making the precise overlay of PET and CT particularly helpful. Similarly, PET/CT can aid in multifocal diseases, such as lymphoma, by providing more exact locations for biopsies and surgery (http://www.cumc.columbia.edu/dept/radiology/pet/p_whatpetct.html).

The scan is preceded by a twelve-hour fast, which is why I'm there first thing in the morning. A technician injects me with the fluorine and I sit still for an hour while the radioactive glucose gets into the cells, at which point I lie still for another twenty-five minutes for the scan itself. I get a kink in my shoulder but manage not to move.

My bone marrow biopsy is another out-of-body experience. I'm drugged for the procedure, which is fine by me as I don't want to be around for anything involving a needle the size of a pencil.

To complete the testing trifecta, I get a MUGA (Multiple Uptake Gated Acquisition) scan. It's a nuclear medicine test to evaluate the function of the heart ventricles and see if they're strong enough to endure what the medical community is about to do to me. I'm injected with radioactive particles and photographed with a gamma camera. Like the other tests I've had so far, this one is painless and mostly involves lying still.

By the end of July I've had enough radioactive procedures to make me glow but the doctors have the data needed to plan my future. For me, a cancer diagnosis is like being told there's a cliff paralleling the path I'm on. At some points they are very close together. I could fall off soon or I could walk on for miles. Either way I don't expect to drop into oblivion or perdition. I think there's another realm of existence just over the edge.

Still, the cliff frightens me.

o   o   o

"Dying is a very dull, dreary affair.
And my advice to you is to have nothing
whatever to do with it."
—Somerset Maughan

CANCER 101

Our word "oncology" comes from the Greek *onkos*, meaning bulk, mass or tumor, and the suffix *logy*, meaning "to poke at." The study of tumors includes diagnosis, therapy, follow-up and palliative care of people with cancer. An MD who specializes in treating cancer is called an oncologist. Susan and I meet mine on Saturday, August 2, at the Memorial Cancer Center.

Dr. Dax Kurbegov wears a shirt and tie; no white coat or excessive formality, which makes it easier to relax. He has a quick smile and ready laugh. He's a well-trained, well-spoken hematologist/oncologist who also happens to be the Medical Director of an award-winning clinic. Nothing like starting at the top!

Based on all the tests, Dr. Dax confirms non-Hodgkin lymphoma, putting me among the more than half-million Americans with this type of cancer. Hodgkin lymphoma, aka Hodgkin disease, is an "eponymous" disease, meaning it's named after the person who first described the condition, in this case British pathologist Thomas Hodgkin. He wrote about what became his namesake in 1832. (Tip: If you're going to have a disease named after you, it's better to be the doctor than the patient.)

It seems strange to have a life-threatening "non" disease. You never hear of non-leukemia or non-melanoma, or of people having non-Alzheimer's (named after Alois Alzheimer) or non-Parkinson's (James Parkinson). Both kinds of lymphoma affect white blood cells called lymphocytes but Hodgkin lymphoma produces an abnormal cell called a Reed-Sternberg cell while non-Hodgkin lymphoma doesn't. The culprit is named after Dorothy Reed Mendenhall and Carl Sternberg. If you want to know why, look it up. I can't do *all* the work.

As it turns out, the non-Hodgkin variety is much more common and spreading at a faster rate in the United States. There are about thirty different forms of NHL and the distinctions are important when it comes to treatment. The Leukemia & Lymphoma Society (LLS) has the following helpful overview:

> Non-Hodgkin lymphoma (NHL) is the term for a diverse group of blood cancers that share a single characteristic—they arise from an injury to the DNA of a lymphocyte progenitor. The damage to the DNA is acquired (occurs after birth) rather than inherited. The altered DNA in one lymphocyte produces a malignant transformation. This transformation results in the uncontrolled and exaggerated growth of the lymphocyte; it gives the malignant lymphocyte and the cells that are formed from its multiplication a survival advantage. The accumulation of those cells results in the tumor masses found in the lymph nodes and other sites in the body.

LLS stats reveal that one American is diagnosed with a blood cancer every four minutes and it kills someone every ten minutes. An estimated 149,990 people in the United States are expected to be diagnosed with leukemia, lymphoma or myeloma in 2013. New cases of these cancers are expected to account for nine percent of the estimated 1,660,290 new cancer cases diagnosed in the United States in 2013. LLS goes on to note there are

» an estimated 694,577 people living with, or in remission from, lymphoma in the United States.
» For NHL, an estimated 529,222 people are living with the disease or are in remission.
» In 2013, there are expected to be 79,030 new cases of lymphoma diagnosed in the United States (9,290 cases of HL, 69,740 cases of NHL).
» In 2013, 20,200 people were expected to die from lymphoma (1,180 from HL, 19,020 from NHL).
» NHL is the seventh most common cancer in the United States, and age-adjusted incidence rose by 82.6 percent from 1975 to 2009.

My disease is at Stage II (out of IV). My bone marrow is unaffected and the cancer has not metastasized—spread elsewhere in my body. I have no other complications and should respond well to chemo.

Toxic Chemo

Chemotherapy chemicals are so toxic they aren't injected into a regular vein but are given through a special port surgically implanted in the chest. So I have to go back to Dr. Dillon on Friday, August 8, for a physical in prep for surgery to be done the following Monday. The first of six rounds of chemotherapy will begin bright and early the following Tuesday morning.

Before starting chemo, the patient is given an overview of the whole procedure. Sharon, an oncology nurse at the clinic, spends several hours teaching me and Susan about RCHOP. That's the regime I'll get once every three weeks for six cycles. I will wind up with more pharmaceuticals in me than a rock star.

We learn that the goal of chemo is to kill part of your body without killing all of you. It involves lethal drugs that do serious damage, hence the side effects. The drugs work by damaging the RNA or DNA that controls cell division. If cells are unable to divide, they die. Healthy cells grow back; hopefully the cancer cells won't.

A hundred years from now chemotherapy may be looked back upon with the same aversion we have to bloodletting today as a barbarous rite of pre-enlightened medicine. For almost 2,000 years concerned physicians drained copious amounts of the vital fluid to relieve their patients of "bad blood."

The practice was supported by the best scientific minds of the time and was based on observation of the body itself, specifically menstruation. None other than the father of medicine, Hippocrates—who gave us the word "cancer"—believed menstruation purged women of bad humors. His most famous student, Galen, began physician-initiated bloodletting in the second century.

Bloodletting was once used to treat cancer, along with everything else from cholera to diabetes, herpes to leprosy, plague to pneumonia, and scurvy to smallpox. The earliest recorded cancer treatment comes from the Egyptians, who used a "fire drill" to cauterize tumors. Medical science lurches forward by trial and error. Even great advances sometimes have unforeseen consequences. A popular theory regarding how AIDS entered the human population posits that it came from chimps whose organs and fluids were used in culturing a strand of oral polio vaccine used in the Congo, the epicenter of the pandemic.

Never mind inadvertent danger, modern chemo causes lots of collateral damage. It's a shotgun that indiscriminately kills both terrorists and hostages. But for many forms of cancer, it's the best weapon we have right now.

Chemo is one of those things in life for which a stunt double would be great. Other experiences where a stand-in would be wonderful are

» childbirth
» IRS audit
» root canal
» prostate exam
» colonoscopy
» (add your least favorite activity here)

Why Me?

While I have asked this question about other things in life, I have not asked it with regard to getting cancer. An estimated 13.7 million Americans with a history of cancer were alive on January 1, 2012, and by January 1, 2022, that number will increase to nearly eighteen million. Why should I expect immunity from this lethal lottery?

"Why" questions can be exercises in futility. While some things are more statistically probable—smokers getting lung cancer, drunk drivers having accidents—others are complete mysteries. *Tour de France* winners get cancer, too, and non-drinkers cause accidents. Bad things happen to good people.

When it comes to individual events, life can be more akin to quantum mechanics than classical physics. Chance sometimes trumps cause and effect. "The race is not to the swift or the battle to the strong, nor does food come to the wise or wealth to the brilliant or favor to the learned; but time and chance happen to them all" (Ecclesiastes 9:11). The more important question is, "How am I going to play the hand I've been dealt?"

Here are five things I recommend if diagnosed with cancer:

1. Read *Anticancer* by David Servan-Schreiber and heed his advice.

2. Clean up your diet in line with *Foods To Fight Cancer* by Richard Beliveau.

3. Exercise regularly—something more than jumping to conclusions and throwing your weight around.

4. Stay engaged; don't withdraw from people. You'll need them now more than ever.

5. Don't wait till you get cancer to start doing these things.

o   o   o

"It would be contrary to the meaning of Providence,
and to the perfection of things, if there were no chance events."
—Thomas Aquinas

IN THE CLINIC

The day prior to my first stint in the chemo clinic I get a "port," aka central venous access device, surgically implanted on the right side of my chest below the collarbone. It's a small round receptacle about the size of a fifty-cent piece into which drugs can be injected. It's placed under the skin with a tube threaded through a blood vessel to just above the heart. Chemo drugs are too caustic for ordinary veins so they have to be injected where the volume is greater and dispersal is faster.

It's an outpatient surgery and only takes about twenty minutes. Still, it's my first time under anesthetic or in an operating room. It won't be my last. I remember bits and pieces of it but not everything Susan says I said.

On Tuesday, August 12, I report to the oncology clinic at Memorial Hospital for my first round of RCHOP chemotherapy, the standard treatment for aggressive lymphoma.

R - Rituximab (aka Rituxan) is a "monoclonal antibody" given as an infusion over several hours. It's an immunotherapy that targets B-cells. Side effects can include infusion reaction, fever, chills, nausea, weakness and headaches. It can also lower platelet and white blood counts, increasing the chance of infection.

C - Cyclophosphamide (aka Cytoxan/Neosar) is a derivative of mustard gas. It slows or stops cell growth. It also lowers the immune system's response to various diseases. Side effects can include nausea, vomiting, bone marrow suppression, mouth sores, diarrhea, bladder irritation, alopecia (hair loss) and lethargy.

H - *Doxorubicin* (trade name Hydroxyldaunorubicin, hence the "H") is an antitumor antibiotic known as "Red Devil" because it turns the urine bright red. Side effects can include nausea, vomiting, neutropenia (decrease in white blood cells) and hair loss. The main danger is heart arrhythmias and congestive heart failure, which is why there's a lifetime cap on the dosage.

O - *Vincristine* (trade name Oncovin, hence the "O") is a "vesicant" that causes extensive tissue damage. It interferes with cell growth, both cancerous and normal. Side effects can include peripheral neuropathy (nerve damage, usually temporary), hyponatremia (an electrolyte disturbance), constipation, hair loss, low blood counts and weight loss.

P - *Prednisolone* (aka Prednisone) is a corticosteroid drug taken orally for the first five days of treatment. It decreases inflammation around tumors by interfering with white blood cells. Side effects can include fluid retention in the face, acne, constipation and mood swings. It can also cause blurred vision, increased thirst, confusion, nervousness and insomnia.

Fortunately most people don't get all these side effects. We'll see how my body reacts and how well my mind can hang on for the ride.

Take a Seat

Once I choose a recliner, I am hooked up to an IV and given Benadryl. A saline drip is also started to keep me hydrated. Next on the menu is Rituxan. Some people have a strong reaction but I tolerate it okay. The Rituxan is given slowly and it's almost 2 p.m. by the time I get the cyclophosphamide. All day I've been guzzling like a camel and peeing like a racehorse. The idea is to flush the toxins out of the body before they damage the liver, kidney and bladder. The nurses have to wear special gloves and garb just to handle the corrosive stuff.

There are about a dozen recliners in the clinic and quite a few people shuffle through during the day. The staff and volunteers do everything to make their "guests" comfortable. Susan is by my side, as she has been throughout my various ordeals. (Unless I'm talking about an actual procedure, you can attach "and Susan" to most uses of "I" and "me.")

I watch the Summer Olympics while I'm being drugged and I think of the comparison between the champions competing in front of the world and the volunteers serving in this oncology clinic. Olympians are made from a unique convergence of circumstances: natural skills, intense training, expert coaching, financial backing and national sponsorship. Volunteers are seldom as richly blessed. They are usually normal people with ordinary abilities and little training. They receive sparse recognition and no financial reward. None of them have ever graced a Wheaties box.

Consider Elaine, who comes to the clinic most Tuesdays. She has a lovely voice and an even lovelier spirit. She's a breast cancer survivor who shares her music and her story with total strangers to encourage them. "You can beat this thing," she says. "I'm living proof!" I requested anything by the Eagles and got a good rendition of "Tequila Sunrise."

Then there's Susan, who wheels by in the afternoon with a warm smile and hot drinks. If she doesn't have it on her cart, she'll get it for you. I order blueberry herbal tea to go along with my Red Devil.

It's thrilling to see Michael Phelps make history. The gymnasts are surreal. Have you ever tried to do an Iron Cross? Treanor and Walsh are unbeatable on sand. But who will be on the pedestals a hundred years from today?

I have no reaction to the first drugs and the ones I get later don't have immediate side effects, so I leave the clinic about 6 p.m. feeling fine, which is surprising given the potency of what they've squirted into me.

o o o

"A 165-pound body consists of about 110 pounds of oxygen, 30 pounds of carbon, 16 pounds of hydrogen, 6 pounds of nitrogen, and 3 pounds of everything else. Basic stuff mostly, the stuff of water and air."
—Chet Raymo

A CLIENT, NOT A PATIENT

I've learned just how expensive cancer drugs can be. Some individual drugs cost as much as $50 thousand to $100 thousand a year—never mind a chemo cocktail! On the other side of the spectrum from designer drugs are natural cures featuring everything from alkaline water to coffee colonics.

Obviously traditional medicine isn't going to embrace alternative medicine or it wouldn't be alternative. Facts are facts and there should be more than anecdotal data to back up the claims of those outside the medical establishment. The debate rages on. I've read information from both perspectives and will try to steer a sane course toward health and recovery.

I won't be able to change the nomenclature of the medical profession but I refer to myself as a client, not a patient. By definition, a patient is "one who receives medical attention or treatment." The archaic meaning was "one who suffers," from the Latin verb meaning "to endure." A client on the other hand is "the party for whom professional services are rendered."

Catch the nuance? A patient is the object of medical care; a client is the subject of medical services. In language as in life, an object is passive, a subject is active.

A patient complies with the experts. A client consults the

experts, then follows what seems the best advice.

A patient might complain but would never contradict an authority. A client will ask questions and weigh alternatives before deciding.

A patient goes where sent and doesn't change doctors or clinics. A client tries to find the best physicians and facilities realistically available.

A patient asks, "What?" A client asks, "Why?"

Being a client takes a lot more work. I have to educate myself about my condition and treatment options. It's a daunting but doable task thanks to the Internet. There are plenty of reputable sites with reliable information the average person can understand.

Oncologists know a shipload more about lymphoma than do its sufferers but they don't know everything. It's impossible to keep up with the tsunami of new information. A dialogue with a well-informed client could suggest new possibilities to a thoughtful physician. I'm not trying to play doctor or impress anyone with my research skills. I'm just trying to understand my cancer and to be proactive in eradicating it. After all, it's my life.

"Civil" War

Since being diagnosed with cancer, I've picked up on the animosity between conventional and alternative approaches to the disease. It can be quite contentious, no doubt because the stakes are so high. The lines are drawn: Western vs. Eastern; big business vs. folk culture; pharmaceuticals vs. herbs; MDs vs. doctors of chiropractic, naturopathy and homeopathy. Both sides in this civil war have their weaknesses and blind spots.

Conventional medicine is misguided when it treats the human body as a machine to be serviced by white-coated mechanics. We are complex creatures who are much more than the sum of our parts. With apologies to René Descartes, our minds do influence our bodies in profound ways. The medical establishment is also remiss in not focusing more on prevention as the first line of defense against disease and in not seeing nutrition as a vital part of treatment.

Alternative medicine is dangerous whenever it touts exotic cure-alls. There are no magic elixirs that can put everything right, even if they do come from a prehistoric valley in Utah (Dr. Wallach's colloidal minerals) or from Himalayan-grown amalaki (Zrii), or from the inner leaf of the Aloe Vera plant (Ambrotose). Proper diet is central to maintaining or restoring good health but not every medical condition can be fixed orally.

Dr. Ralph Moss offers sage advice in his CancerDecisions.com newsletter:

> Cancer is a complex disease. It requires professional help. Regardless of the sometimes uncaring attitude of certain errant members of the medical profession, one should not reject everything that conventional medicine has to offer in favor of a regimen discovered on the Internet. The answer is not simply to construct a do-it-yourself program but to find expert and sympathetic guidance in the rapidly expanding realm of complementary oncology.

I like the term "complementary." It is built into the approach of the Memorial Cancer Center where I'm a client. They proclaim, "By integrating complementary therapies with traditional medicine, we will take a holistic approach to cancer medicine that addresses patients' physical, emotional and spiritual needs."

A dose of humility is in order for professionals of every stripe. When it comes to medicine no one has all the answers; everyone is still practicing.

Health in Motion

As life goes on around me, I definitely feel like the odd man out. We Americans are obsessed with health: health clubs, health foods, health care. Good health is at the core of our individual and national self-image. But what does it mean to be healthy? Clotaire Rapaille, author of *The Culture Code*, has done worldwide research on cultural differences. He's uncovered the disparate views of love, sex, food, success, beauty, health and scores of other ideals that are based on a shared history and lead to a common worldview.

Rapaille points out that America "is a nation of doers. For us, health and wellness means being able to complete your mission … If Americans believe they are strong enough to act, then they are healthy. Their greatest fear about being sick is their inability to do things. The code word for health and wellness in America is *movement*."

I'm all American when it comes to my health. What I hate about cancer and all other illnesses are the restrictions they impose. Being healthy means being free to do what I want physically—within reason. Being sick means being hobbled by weakness and limitations.

When it comes to doctors, Rapaille notes that our code word is "hero" because these white-coats rescue us and restore our abilities. Our code word for nurses is "mother" because they are with us in difficult times and see to our best interests. No wonder nursing consistently tops the list of our most respected professions.

Unlike doctors and nurses, hospitals inspire a sense of foreboding. According to Rapaille, the code for hospitals in America is "processing plant." Medicinal and mechanical processes overwhelm the care-giving element. If health is movement, then hospitals are decidedly unhealthy places. Once admitted, you are webbed down by tubes and cords. When you do move about, you are tethered to a pole. You can't even leave under your own power but must be wheeled to the curb. The only institution with a more aggressive confinement policy is the penal system.

I'm thankful for all the healthcare advances that have come through hospitals but I'm also thankful I haven't had to be hospitalized yet. I'd like to keep it that way. Other than some bone aches, I feel pretty good, relatively speaking. But I got a sober reminder of cancer's pernicious temperament the last time I was at the clinic to have my blood drawn. I read an article in the Memorial Clinic newsletter about the Thomas House:

> The Thomas House is a new lodging resource for Memorial cancer patients traveling to Colorado Springs for treatment. It is a comfortable two-bedroom apartment within walking distance of Memorial Hospital. … This wonderful venture is the brainchild of the sister of a former cancer patient, Bill Thomas, a Colorado Springs Police Department detective. … There is no monetary charge to patients but a donation of $10 per night is appreciated for those who are able to contribute.

The generosity of this act touched me, but not as deeply as the event that caused it. Bill Thomas died of non-Hodgkin lymphoma.

o   o   o

"Someone once asked me if my dream was
to live on in the hearts of people, and I said
I would like to live on in my apartment."
—Woody Allen

FARTS AND FALLOUT

I went in for my second round of chemo on Tuesday, September 2. My daughter, Julie, brought me in and Susan took over at lunch. They know I need adult supervision at all times. I sit in a corner chair because it has more room. It's like being in a library with IV poles. My nurse is Mary Beth and she's wonderful, like all the clinic staff I've met so far. I have my phone and laptop and am able to stay busy.

By 1:10 p.m. I finish one bag and have three more to go. I get a booster of Zofran to prevent nausea and other reactions. At 2:00 p.m. I start the Red Devil, the stuff they can't let touch your skin or anything else because it's a vesicant. It's also hard on the kidneys and you have to get it out of your system as soon as possible, hence the copious drinking. At 3:50 p.m. Mary Beth hangs my last bag, which means I finish earlier than last time.

I've come up with a new version of a popular TV show I call Survivor: Chemo. To qualify, contestants must have a white blood count above 3.5 K/mcl and not be afraid of needles. They would have a series of toxic drugs injected into them, after which they would compete at various tasks like:

» correctly pronouncing the concoctions they're on (e.g.

cyclophosphamide or doxorubicin);
» pole racing to the bathroom;
» peeing orange, darkest color wins;
» eating hospital food;
» sleeping through the night at any time during the next week.

Contestants could be voted out of the clinic for:
» allergic reactions (this gets you carted off to the emergency room);
» bad-mouthing the pharmacist;
» excessive shedding;
» complaining about the magazine selection;
» watching Fox News on the TVs above their recliners;
» screaming during the removal of chest hair via postcard-sized bandages (for those who *have* chest hair).

There is no immunity in Survivor: Chemo as the drugs wipe it out. A contestant who makes it through six or more rounds earns the right to be called a Survivor.

Nothing "Side" about It

The "side" effects of chemo soon take center stage in my life. Two of the most noticeable are chemo farts and hair loss. While not mentioned often in the literature and blogs I've read, fetid fumes are a byproduct of cancer treatment. Not surprising since one of my chemo drugs is cyclophosphamide, a derivative of mustard gas. The foul odor of normal flatus mainly results from
» low molecular weight fatty acids such as butyric acid (rancid butter smell);
» reduced sulfur compounds such as hydrogen sulfide (rotten egg smell);

» carbonyl sulfides that are the result of protein breakdown.

Pharmaceutically enhanced flatulence is in a whole other class from everyday gas. It is wicked deadly and should be avoided, especially by pregnant women and nursing mothers. If you encounter it, hold your breath and back out of the room. The perpetrator will understand. One solution would be the airtight underwear with a replaceable charcoal filter invented by Chester Weimer of nearby Pueblo, Colorado. Another is just to grin, closed lipped, and bear it.

My hair started falling out last week. While driving home from the library I scratched my head at a stoplight and came away with wolf-man fingers. Ironically I had just made an appointment for a haircut, which I had to cancel. It doesn't take long to go from *alopecia aerate* to *alopecia totalis*. Over the next few days I started shedding like a Shih Tzu, so I decided on a preemptive strike. I had my son-in-law, Alan, shave my head. I made it a family affair so the grandkids wouldn't be scared the next time they saw me. Still, it freaked out my grandson Jason for a few days.

I buy a hat but don't wear it all the time. I want to get enough sun so that I look like a brown egg instead of a white one. For Halloween next month I can wear an orange sheet and be a Tibetan monk or a green sweatshirt with a pillow in back and go as a turtle.

In addition to falling hair, my white blood count (WBC) is dropping. It gets so low that I was grounded for a while. No restaurants. No wedding on Saturday. No church on Sunday—too many germs about for someone in my state of caducity. The normal WBC range is from 3.5 to 10.6 K/mcl. My count is 3.3 and that means my immune system is in the crapper.

o   o   o

Blood test, sans needle. True or False:

1. There are half a million white blood cells in every drop of human blood.
2. White blood cells live a few weeks but red blood cells live about four months.
3. Your white blood count is usually lower in the morning than the afternoon.
4. White blood cells are formed from bone marrow stem cells.
5. Smoking may cause an increase in white blood cells.
6. White blood cells are colorless because they don't contain hemoglobin.
7. About seven percent of your body weight is blood (7-9 quarts in the average adult).
8. When white blood cells die they are destroyed by other white blood cells.
9. Dr. Spock's blood was green because it contained copper.
10. There is no blood in Blood Pudding.

(All the above are true except #10.)

FLAT AS A SHADOW

Between rounds three and four of chemo I get another PET scan. It's supposed to be predictive of the eighteen-month outcome in patients with intermediate and aggressive NHL and should help in the identification of patients who would benefit from more intensive treatment. Mine comes back clean. It shows some slightly enlarged lymph nodes where the tumors used to be, but this could be scar tissue. The term "unofficial remission" is used. "Remission" means there's no sign of cancer in my body; "unofficial" is because this has to be confirmed by a follow-up PET scan after I finish chemo.

Emotionally, I feel like I'm in a beautiful clearing, yet still with a long way to go until I'm out of the woods. Cancer can return, especially in the first two years after treatment. According to the Leukemia & Lymphoma Society, the five-year relative survival rate for NHL has risen from thirty-one percent among Caucasians in the 1960s to sixty-nine percent for all races from 1999 to 2006. It looks like I've been effectively drugged into the fortunate two-thirds of the equation.

Physically, I feel a wedge of weariness from my shoulders to my groin. My solar plexus aches. My posture is a C-. But at least my sharp is still mind (sic). I've experienced no nausea so far, thank God, but the prednisone messes with my sleep and leaves me both tired and fatigued. There's a difference you know. Tiredness is a normal part of life. It results from exertion and stress and is usually fixed by a good night's sleep. Fatigue is a whole-body lack of energy signaling a decreased capacity or complete inability to function normally. It is not relieved by sleep.

A "tiredness continuum" might look like this:

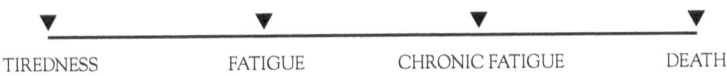

| TIREDNESS | FATIGUE | CHRONIC FATIGUE | DEATH |

"It is important to recognize the difference between tiredness and fatigue, because fatigue is a marker that the body is not able to keep up," says Dr. Karin Olson of the Alberta Heritage Foundation for Medical Research. Dr. Olsen points out that individuals who are tired still have a fair bit of energy, so although they may feel forgetful and impatient and experience gradual heaviness or weakness in muscles following work, this is often alleviated by rest. Fatigue, on the other hand, is characterized by difficulty concentrating, anxiety, a gradual decrease in stamina, difficulty sleeping, increased sensitivity to light and the limiting of social activities once viewed as important.

One of the more common side effects of cancer and its treatment is cancer-related fatigue (CRF). It can occur suddenly; it does not result from activity or exertion; and sleep does not relieve it. It may continue even after treatment is complete. There are some practical ways to deal with tiredness, fatigue and CRF, but I'm too bushed to type them out. Visit the Cleveland Clinic Web page on CRF for helpful tips on how to cope.

There are other, less serious annoyances that have collected like dryer lint and make it harder for me to live normally:

» I've lost my taste for coffee, a habit I've cultivated my entire adult life. And I just got a French press for my birthday.

» I'm no longer interested in my daily glass of wine, which is fine because alcohol is *verboten* during chemo.

» I have a yucky taste in my mouth and queasiness in my stomach most of the time. Not quite nausea but not quite normal.

» The port in my chest sticks out like an acorn. My grandkids bump it when I pick them up and the shoulder belt in the car catches on it.

» Because my sleep pattern is messed up, my energy level is worn down. It's like someone let the air out of my tires and I'm running on the rims.

There are other changes. I've given up shaking hands. When I walk into church I think of how we station greeters to collect germs from everyone entering and to spread the little buggers throughout the community. I've also given up keeping the household budget balanced. The medical column refuses to stay in line. It's looting and pillaging its neighbors. I take solace from the words of that great economist Sinbad: "It's only money; they print more of it every day."

Sleepless in Colorado

Insomnia is the most persistent side effect of my chemo. I can't go to sleep without taking a couple of pills. Not wanting to become dependent, I try to go without them once every few nights, without success. Just my luck, I'll finish chemo and have to enter rehab to get off sleeping pills.

Joking—I hope—aside, I'm very thankful for the pills. They make the subsequent rounds of chemo more tolerable than the first. There's a reason why sleep deprivation is a universal form of torture. In the short term it causes concentration and memory impairment and irritability. More sleepless nights can lead to slurred speech, tremors, hypertension and hallucinations. Long-term effects can include weakened immune system, heart disease, depression, mental illness and even death. You will die faster from sleep deprivation than starvation.

One hypothesis is that deprivation mimics the effects of selective serotonin reuptake inhibitors (SSRI). Another is that REM sleep is essential for blocking neurotransmitters and allowing the neurotransmitter receptors to rest and regain sensitivity, which leads to improved regulation of mood and increased learning ability. If your brain can't rejuvenate, you deteriorate.

Matthew Walker, Director of the Sleep and Neuroimaging Lab at the University of California, Berkeley, discovered a disconnect in the brains of sleep-deprived people between the amygdala and the frontal lobe, the region controlling rational thought and decision-making. This results in emotional responses not being kept in check by the more logical seat of reasoning. The same problem is found in people with psychiatric disorders.

Translation: Sleeplessness can make you nuts!

Or help you become more spiritual. The Desert Fathers denied themselves sleep as a spiritual discipline and some historians believe coffee's popularity was enhanced by Muslim mystics who used it to pull all-night devotionals.

Unfortunately, it hasn't worked that way for me yet.

o   o   o

"The worst thing in the world
is to try to sleep and not to."
—F. Scott Fitzgerald

BLESSED

'm in the oncology clinic today, November 4, for my fifth round of chemo. "Blessed" isn't a word usually associated with chemo but I feel blessed to have the medical care I do. I'm blessed by the technology and those who lovingly administer it. Nurses don't wear hats anymore, but if they did, oncology nurses would be in green berets. They are on the front lines in the war on cancer. What makes them want to work daily with sick and dying people? I asked two of the ones I've gotten to know over the past few months.

Anne has been an oncology nurse for seven years. She got interested in this branch of nursing after caring for her mother-in-law who died of lung cancer. Her father also died of cancer. "The patients are so awesome," Anne says. "I try to be friendly with them but not to become friends because it's hard to lose one. You can't do your job if you're grieving all the time."

Michelle took eighteen years off from nursing to raise and homeschool five children. Now she's back in the oncology clinic at Memorial Hospital. "The hard part is dealing with what you can't control," Michelle says. "But the patients are great because they are much more engaged in their condition and eager to cooperate. They're my heroes."

Nurses are my heroes. The essence of what they do is captured in one of my favorite cartoons. It shows a man standing before a concerned St. Peter who is studying his clipboard. The new arrival says, "Sorry I'm late; I had great nurses."

Life on a T-Shirt

I see a few cancer-related T-shirts in the clinic. Nobel laureate Leon Lederman once said, "My ambition is to live to see all of physics reduced to a formula so elegant and simple that it will fit easily on the front of a T-shirt." He was talking about the Big TOE (Theory of Everything) and his comment inspired a book I read by Dan Falk on the current state of physics, *Universe on a T-Shirt*.

Understanding the entire universe is beyond my pay grade but I've always looked for elegant and simple explanations of how life works. Distilling truth is a venerable tradition. Think of the proverbs in the Old Testament or the sayings of Jesus in the New: "Render unto Caesar …, What shall it profit a man …, Greater love has no man than this …."

The T-shirt template requires principles that are profound, pithy and portable. Words that are wise, witty and wearable. Maxims that are memorable, meaty and mobile. Sayings that are sagacious, sharp and salable. (I could go on and on; just ask my kids.) Here are a few quips worthy of being worn in cotton. My favorite cancer T-shirts are:

Does This Shirt Make My Head Look Bald?

I have Chemo Brain. What's Your Excuse?

I'm a Lymphomaniac!

Save the Boobies!

o o o

"Sometimes life is like a B-movie.
You don't want to leave in the middle,
but you don't want to see it again."
—Ted Turner

BETTER LIVING THROUGH DRUGS

P harmaceuticals are risky business. Having them prescribed and monitored by a doctor is a safeguard but it doesn't make them safe. I choose to be repeatedly injected with toxic chemotherapy because, after doing some research, I believe it affords me the best chance of staying alive, but the price I'll pay won't be fully known for some time.

My next drug challenge after chemo will be weaning myself off the various sleeping pills I've been snorking since August. I don't know how long it will take my brain to get chemically balanced—as if my brain has ever been balanced—or for me to get a normal night's sleep. I don't expect the transition to be easy. In her book, *Another Day in the Frontal Lobe*, neurosurgeon Katrina Firkin notes:

> Anything strong enough to help you is strong enough to hurt you. No treatment, at least no worthwhile treatment, comes without risk. Even natural supplements, if you take unnaturally large amounts, can have untoward effects. … There are plenty of medications that work wonders without us having a clear idea as to how or why they work. To me, that means there are probably other things those drugs are doing that we may not

expect. It would be unlikely for a drug to have one and only one effect on the body. That's not how the body works. One physiological mechanism can mediate numerous different functions. One natural chemical, blocked or enhanced by a certain drug, may have dozens of different targets. Those targets are probably not all figured out yet.

One drug I haven't mentioned yet is Neulasta. Every time I get chemo I have to return to the clinic the day after for a shot of it. A strong chemo regime results in a low white-blood count, which increases the risk of infections. Neulasta is a white-cell booster that, along with the Rituxan given at the start of chemo, has dramatically improved survivability, especially for those of us with non-Hodgkin lymphoma.

Clinical Trial

I have greatly benefited from the experiences of those who have had cancer before me and I want to help others who will be diagnosed with the disease in the future. That's why I asked Dr. Dax about any clinical trials I could join.

Clinical trials are "biomedical or health-related research studies in human beings that follow a pre-defined protocol. It turns out there's one underway for NHL involving enzastaurin, which sounds like a citizen of a Central Asian country but is really a new drug showing promise in suppressing tumor cell growth and inhibiting tumor-induced angiogenesis.

Clinical trials come in four phases. This one is a Phase III trial, which means enzastaurin has already been extensively tested. Now the pharmaceutical company and the FDA want a large-scale trial to gain a more thorough understanding of its effectiveness and to determine the range of possible adverse reactions. While some doctors make money on trials, there's usually no financial incentive for the patients, other than free drugs. Involvement is voluntary and participants can withdraw at any time. There are potential pros and cons to consider before enrolling:

Upsides:

» getting early access to new treatments and promising pharmaceuticals
» enjoying meticulous care and state-of-the-art monitoring
» contributing to medical knowledge that could save thousands
» gaining cool super powers like X-ray vision or spidey sense

Downsides:

» receiving no benefit, either because you're in the control group given placebos or because the drug doesn't work
» experiencing unpleasant side effects or serious adverse reactions
» investing the extra time and effort it takes to follow the sometimes complex protocols
» having your body glow in the dark

Not just anyone can qualify for a clinical trial; you have to be "special." You don't want to be *too* special, though, as in having a rare medical condition named after you.

First doctor: "Poor guy; he's got Hamel's Disease."

Second doctor: "You sure he wasn't hit by a bus?"

First doctor: "I believe the autopsy will prove I'm right."

International Prognosis Index

A few days after asking, I learn that I don't qualify for the enzastaurin clinical trial. My IPI is too low, which turns out to be a good thing. IPI stands for International Prognosis Index. It was developed fifteen years ago by oncologists as a clinical tool to help predict the prognosis of patients with aggressive non-Hodgkin lymphoma. In the Index, one point is assigned for each of these risk factors:

» age greater than sixty years
» stage III or IV disease
» elevated serum LDH (lactate dehydrogenase)
» ECOG/Zubrod performance status of 2, 3, or 4
» more than 1 extranodal site

The total points correlate to the following risk groups:

» low risk (0-1 points): 5-year survival of 73 percent
» low-intermediate risk (2 points): 5-year survival of 51 percent
» high-intermediate risk (3 points): 5-year survival of 43 percent
» high risk (4-5 points): 5-year survival of 26 percent

These correlations may be out of date in that they are based on data prior to the widespread use of Rituxan, which has improved the outcomes for B-cell lymphoma patients. After finishing six rounds of chemo there's no sign of active cancer. My IPI is 1, which means I have a low risk of return and a high chance of going into remission. But there are no guarantees. If the cancer does come back, the next course of action would be a bone marrow transplant and I don't want to contemplate that possibility. I just want to bask in the initial success of treatment.

"Bask" isn't the right word; "crapulence" is a better term to describe how I feel. Crapulence was in the dictionary long before Monty Burns used it on *The Simpsons*. It's now in my vocabulary as the perfect word to describe chemo and its aftermath. Crapulence is sickness caused by excessive eating or drinking (or drugging). My side effects could have been much worse. Still, chemo is about as fun as a field tracheotomy or removing your own teeth with a rock *a la* Tom Hanks in *Cast Away*. The upside is the drugs appear to have napalmed my cancer for the time being. I'll know more in January.

o   o   o

"I believe in pretense, I believe in elegance and glamour;
and I believe that sometimes you just have
to look reality in the eye and deny it."
—Garrison Keillor

SLEEP ON IT

One of the practical comforts I've had during my bout with cancer is a good bed. A great bed actually, which has helped me cope with insomnia. My thinking on sleep surfaces has changed over the years and reflects what I consider to be my growing maturity. As a new Christian I slept on the floor in a sleeping bag next to my bed. At the time I was associated with a group known as the Plymouth Brethren. (My thesaurus gives that name as a synonym for "ascetic.") No one told me to do this; I just picked up that denying the body was part of pleasing the Lord. Susan threw out my sleeping bag when we got married. She wasn't as spiritual.

Years later when our first bed wore out I bought a new one. It had a pillow top and I felt so guilty about the extra padding that I returned the bed the next day and bought one for $100 less, much to Susan's consternation. Last spring I sprung for our third bed in thirty-four years, not counting a short fling with a leaky waterbed. I shelled out for a Sleep Number bed. At first I balked at spending so much on a glorified air mattress but it's been worth it. Susan heartily agrees.

"Jesus wouldn't own a Sleep Number bed," my younger self might scold. But there are lots of things I own that Jesus didn't, all of which make my life easier than his: a computer, a smart phone, a microwave oven, a toothbrush. While I don't know what he slept on, I do think he slept more than I do, probably retiring and rising with the sun.

A good bed is a key to good health. Many studies show the correlation between quality of sleep and quality of life, such as "Top 10 Health Benefits of a Good Night's Sleep" on About.com. Quantity of sleep is also important. According to a piece on WebMD, "Studies show an increased mortality risk for those reporting less than either six or seven hours per night. One study found that reduced sleep time is a greater mortality risk than smoking, high blood pressure and heart disease."

Bed is where we head when we're sick and tired. It's where we pass a third of our lives. It's where we make some of our happiest memories. It's where we conceive the children who will care for us in our dotage and we want them to be warm, softhearted people. So why is it that we skimp when it comes to cost? Americans probably spend twenty times more on our cars than our beds, yet we spend a tenth of the time behind the wheel as between the sheets. How convoluted is that!

The moral of this bedtime story is don't shortchange yourself; invest in a good night's sleep. In his book, *The Thing About Life Is That One Day You'll Be Dead*, David Shields gives the following stats:

> On average, infants sleep 20 hours a day, 1-year-olds sleep 13 hours a day, teenagers sleep 9 hours, 40-year-olds sleep 7 hours, 50-year-olds sleep 6 hours, and people 65 and older sleep 5 hours. ... By age 65, an unbroken night's sleep is rare; 20 percent of the night consists of lying awake.

Mellow Melatonin

Buying a new bed is an expensive sleep tip, so here's a cheaper one: melatonin. Melatonin is a hormone produced deep in the brain by our pineal gland (believed by Descartes and others to be the location of the soul). It helps regulate our circadian rhythms, including sleep. We make less melatonin as we age, so taking a supplement can help keep life in balance.

The Mayo Clinic reports that "the weight of scientific evidence does suggest that melatonin decreases the time it takes to fall asleep, increases the feeling of sleepiness, and may increase the duration of sleep." Melatonin has been shown to help with jet lag and suggested to help "delay the spread of cancer, strengthen the immune system, or slow the aging process. But these areas need further research." Indeed, one overview of melatonin studies concludes that melatonin isn't effective in *any* of the instances I quote above, so go figure.

What is true is that melatonin is inexpensive and presumed safe for short-term use. Here are some other uses for melatonin, but you didn't hear them from me:

» For a good night's rest, sprinkle it on the supper of an overly amorous spouse.
» To stand out at work, dissolve it in the coffee pot and bring your own brew.
» For parental peace of mind, add it to the punch served at all school dances.
» To enhance a long plane flight, sneak it into the drink of a talkative seatmate (but don't let the sky marshal see you).

o   o   o

Sleep Trivia:
» The record for the longest period without sleep is 18 days, 21 hours, 40 minutes during a rocking-chair marathon.
» Seventeen hours of sustained wakefulness leads to a decrease in performance equivalent to a blood alcohol level of 0.05%.
» A new baby typically results in 400 to 750 hours of lost sleep

for parents in the first year.

» Americans average 6.9 hours of sleep on weeknights and 7.5 hours per night on weekends.

» REM sleep occurs in bursts totaling about two hours a night, usually beginning about ninety minutes after falling asleep.

RECOVERING LYMPHOMANIAC

On Sunday, January 24, 2009, the Hamel family has a party to celebrate Julie's twenty-seventh birthday and my clean scans since completing chemo. I'm now considered to be in remission. The American Cancer Society defines remission:

> A period of time when the cancer is responding to treatment or is under control. In a complete remission, all the signs and symptoms of the disease disappear. It is also possible for a patient to have a partial remission in which the cancer shrinks but does not completely disappear. Remissions can last anywhere from several weeks to many years. Complete remissions may continue for years and be considered cures.

My symptoms are gone, along with the grapefruit-sized abdominal tumor. My energy and appetite have returned, along with my hair. But since lymphoma has a fairly high return rate, I will be closely monitored for the next two years. I can't use the good "C" word (cured) for five years. After that, my chances of getting cancer again are statistically the same as anyone else's, which in the Western world isn't very good news.

No one is cancer free; our bodies make millions of defective cells. I am, however, now among the tumor free, for which I am extremely grateful to God, to my family, to the medical community at Memorial Health System and to all those who have prayed for and helped me along the way. I'm not completely out of the woods but I'm in the clear today and that's the most any of us can say.

Lymphos Anonymous

Hello, my name is Mike and I'm a recovering lymphomaniac. It's been six weeks since my last chemo binge and I'm working hard at staying healthy. As a lympho, I don't have as much energy as I used to, so I've shortened the typical twelve-step recovery program by half:

1. I admitted I was *not* powerless over my disease—cancer can't always be controlled but it can be attacked.
2. I came to believe that a Power greater than myself could restore me to health—and did!
3. I made a decision to turn my life over to the care of God and oncologists as I understood them—with help from Google.
4. I made a searching physical inventory of my habits, listing all substances that had harmed me and determining to avoid them as much as possible—without becoming an anchorite.
5. I sought through prayer and meditation to improve my conscious contact with God—still working on it.
6. Having had a physical restoration as a result of these steps, I tried to encourage others to practice these principles—hence this book.

Recovery starts with self but it's not a self-help program. We need the good graces of others to survive. And without others, who would want to?

Exit Interview

On February 4, I have my survivor checkup with John Himberger,

NP. We go over my medical history and blood work. Then he gives me a physical and pronounces me fit as a ukulele, except that my triglycerides and cholesterol are high. I'll continue to get PET/CT scans in the months ahead to see if my NHL returns. The chemo that stopped it might also make me susceptible to leukemia and other bone marrow disorders down the road. But for now my life is returning to normal, if there is such a thing. I'm back to running and eating and sleeping like I was before cancer—even better when it comes to diet. My next goal is getting back to work fulltime.

In keeping with my newfound health I get "de-ported" the next morning. Dr. Dillon removes the chemo port he installed last August. A battle scar from my war with lymphoma becomes a third nipple.

Monday, February 9, is my thirty-fifth wedding anniversary. Susan and I tied the knot in 1974; the year that saw Patty Hearst kidnapped, President Nixon resign and Muhammad Ali regain the world heavyweight title. The average cost of a new house was $34,900; the average annual income was $13,900; a mid-size new car cost about $3,750 and a gallon of gas was fifty-five cents.

The traditional gift for a thirty-fifth anniversary is coral. The modern gift is jade. I can give Susan neither this year but I can give her something more rare and precious: My unique and undying love.

o　　o　　o

"A successful marriage requires falling in love many times,
always with the same person."
—Mignon McLaughlin

PART II
RELAPSE AND TRANSPLANT
MARCH – AUGUST 2009

"If you can't go around it, over it, or through it,
you had better negotiate with it."
—Ashleigh Brilliant

TROUBLE IN THE REGION

I don't have long to celebrate my return to normalcy. My February 24 PET scan shows swelling in two lymph nodes in the same region as my earlier tumor. Not good news but hopefully not as bad as it sounds. There could be other causes of the inflammation. I'll need to get another biopsy and review the results with Dr. Dax. No sense getting stressed over possibilities in the mean time. Jesus said, "Do not worry about tomorrow, for tomorrow will worry about itself. Each day has enough trouble of its own."

While near the hospital for my PET scan, I drop by the chemo clinic to hug the nurses. These caring professionals work against the odds and experience more loss than most people. It's important for their patients—I mean clients—to come back once in a while and say, "Thanks for all you did. I'm still alive because of you."

We all need to be appreciated; it's food for the soul and oil for the gears of civilization. And as with most other virtues, it is better to give than to receive.

Can you think of someone who has been a blessing to you and who deserves a thank you hug? A parent, spouse, friend, boss, pastor, neighbor? Move that earned embrace to the top of your To Do list. If the worthy party isn't within arm's reach, make a call or send an email.

Don't put it off. In the book, *Life Lessons*, Elizabeth Kubler-Ross and David Kessler tell the story of a woman whose husband died in his sleep at age forty-four. This heartbreaking experience taught her not to take relationships, people or time for granted:

> I looked back at our lives and saw everything so differently. That was our last kiss, our last meal, our last vacation, our last hug. … I understand that Kevin was a gift I could keep for a while but not forever. This is true for everyone I meet. Knowing this makes me take in these moments and people even more.

You can never be too thankful for others but you can be too thoughtless to express it.

It's Back!

We have about five hundred to seven hundred lymph nodes spread throughout our bodies. These are organs, not glands. They filter out and eliminate dead bacteria, viruses and other sloughed off tissue from the lymphatic fluid. Infections and other problems—including cancer—can cause nodes to expand, a condition known as lymphadenopathy. People with persistent localized lymphadenopathy, or those who have risk factors for malignancy, should undergo a biopsy.

A biopsy is the removal of cells or tissues for examination. On Thursday, March 9, I get my fourth one, a fine-needle aspiration of my once cancerous lymph node. It turns out my lymphoma is back. Actually the cancer never left; it was just suppressed by the chemo. It is considered a "relapsed disease" and I will be headed for salvage therapy. That's what they call it—look it up. Salvage therapy is "treatment that is given after the cancer has not responded to other treatments."

The medical community really should do a better job with

their nomenclature. "Relapsed" is bad enough, but "salvage"? That's what you do to wrecked cars and sunken ships. Although to be fair, salvage used as a noun means, "something saved from destruction or waste and put to further use."

I can live with that.

The quick return indicates what's called "refractory" disease rather than a relapse, which is a return after remission. The usual approach to refractory DLBCL is high-dose chemotherapy and autologous stem cell transplant (ASCT), aka a bone marrow transplant. My own stem cells will be harvested and used, no donors or embryos involved. Stem cells are made in the bone marrow and mature into red blood cells, white blood cells and platelets. When they go rogue and produce defective or cancerous cells, one way to stop them is to reboot the bone marrow with a transplant of healthy cells.

I have to have my port put back in and undergo more chemo in preparation for the transplant that will be done at the Rocky Mountain Cancer Center in Denver. I'll know more after I meet with their transplant team.

o   o   o

"Being defeated is often a temporary condition.
Giving up is what makes it permanent."
—Marlene von Savant

TRANSPLANT PREP

$\int$ usan and I drive to Denver on Wednesday, March 18, to meet Dr. Mark Brunvand, the bowtie-wearing transplant hematologist at Rocky Mountain Cancer Center. He is bursting with energy and information. He looks me in the eye when he talks and makes sure he's answered my questions before he moves on. And I've got questions. Before our meeting I did some boning up on bone marrow transplants. BMTs can cure a significant percentage of patients who undergo them. Those who had a good response to initial therapy are the most likely to have a good outcome. There are two types:

Allogeneic: Where donor cells are used. This type has a high probability of curing the patient but is also very dangerous. About twenty to thirty percent of patients die during this procedure and many have severe side effects afterward, which is why it's only used about twenty-five percent of the time with lymphoma patients.

Autologous: Where the patient's own cells are used. This type is very safe (two-percent death rate) but does not have as high a long-term survival rate as allogeneic transplants. Cells are collected before treatment; the person gets high-dose chemo and/or radiation to kill the bone marrow; then the cells are re-infused to repopulate the marrow.

I'm scheduled for an autologous transplant.

If You Have Cancer ...

... why use your own cells in a transplant? This is one of my biggest questions. Dr. Brunvand explained the reasons but I later found this simpler explanation on the NHL Cyberfamily Web site:

> You might think this sounds strange since the patient already has cancer. However there are two characteristics of NHL that are important to understand. First the patient who has NHL has cancer of the white blood cells that circulate in the lymphatic system. Therefore very few if any cancer cells are in the blood. Second, the apheresis procedure collects only stem cells not white blood cells. In theory there should not be any risk of collecting any cancer cells, but unfortunately theory and fact don't quite match. .... And although NHL does not normally circulate in the blood there are always a few roaming cancer cells in the blood. This means that there is a pretty good risk of getting some cancer cells in the stem cell harvest.

In preparation for more chemo and the transplant, I get another type of port inserted into my chest on Friday by my old friend Dr. Dillon. It's a central venous catheter (CVC) called a Hickman line. The catheter is surgically inserted into a vein in the neck or chest and passed under the skin. The end sticks through the skin and is used for injecting medicines into the body.

The Hickman I get is called a triluminal catheter because it has three tails. It's a formidable piece of hardware to be dangling from one's chest but it is essential equipment for a transplant. It can remain in place for extended periods and saves wear and tear on the arm veins during chemo. But it isn't risk free as the line is subject to infection and blood clots. Preventing this requires regular flushing with an anticoagulant called heparin. (You don't want to know the details of how heparin is made from pig intestine or cow lung.)

I also get an antiemetic patch on my upper arm that's the new gold standard in nausea control. It contains granisetron, a recently approved drug in a class of medications called 5-HT3 antagonists. It works by blocking the production of serotonin, which can trigger nausea and vomiting. This is just the baseline; I'll get other medications as needed in the hospital.

All this gives the impression I'm headed for some kick-ass chemo, but killing cancer at its genetic roots is deadly business. The goal is to put me in remission so that clean stem cells can be harvested for my transplant.

Take No Prisoners!

o   o   o

"'Tis not in mortals to command success,
but we'll do more ... we'll deserve it."
—Joseph Addison

REFLECTIONS ON BEING TERMINAL

Every time a cancer treatment is tried and fails—in my case RCHOP chemo—the odds aren't as good the next time around. Almost sixty percent of NHL patients who have RCHOP chemotherapy go into remission, so I didn't make the cut on that one. And about thirty-two to fifty-two percent of those who undergo an autologous transplant make it to the five-year survivability mark. We'll see how I do.

To put this reality into an everyday metaphor, we are all making our way toward the checkout lanes in the supermarket of life. Some people shuffle behind long-lived ancestors with good genes while others suddenly find ourselves in the "10 Items or Fewer" line and closer to the exit.

It can be a shock to wind up in the express lane earlier than anticipated, which for Americans is any age shy of one hundred. But everyone has to leave the building eventually. We all know this, and yet consumerism keeps us absorbed in the moment—until someone crashes into our cart; we slip in the soap aisle or we get a bad chicken salad sandwich in the deli. That's when we're reminded of our mortality.

Having non-Hodgkin lymphoma puts me in a shorter queue than my peers but I know enough not to be fooled by mere geometry.

The shortest line isn't always the fastest moving. When we hear the diagnosis "cancer," the next word we think of is "terminal." Then we want to know "How long do I have?" and we'll sooner than later find a survival graph for our type of cancer. This graph plots a survival curve on an x-y axis showing the number of patients and the amount of time they live. A survival curve can't be reduced to a single number such as the "median" survival or the "overall" survival rate (OS = five years), but this is exactly what everyone looks for.

This rush to data can do more harm than good. Consider the experience of the noted biologist Stephen Jay Gould, who was diagnosed with a rare and serious abdominal mesothelioma in 1982. After surgery, he went in search of his own survival graph:

> As soon as I could walk, I made a beeline for Harvard's Countway medical library and punched mesothelioma into the computer's bibliographic search program. ... The literature couldn't have been more brutally clear: mesothelioma is incurable, with a median mortality of only eight months after discovery.
>
> What does "median mortality of eight months" signify in our vernacular? I suspect that most people, without training in statistics, would read such a statement as "I will probably be dead in eight months"—the very conclusion that must be avoided, since it isn't so, and since attitude matters so much.

Gould used his knowledge as a tool in his successful fight against cancer. He lived for another twenty years, beating the eight-month death sentence thirty times over. He shared his insights on statistics in the article, "The Median Isn't the Message," which has been an encouragement to me and countless others.

Lies, Damned Lies, and Statistics

Dr. Servan-Schreiber reminds us that, "Statistics are information, not condemnation." And Mark Twain used to say there were "lies, damned lies, and statistics." Still, having *any* number put on the right side of our lifeline is a reminder that our shopping days are numbered. It makes us stare into our carts to see what we've collected so far. Things don't count. Nothing physical ever leaves the store. All items here are for rent only. (Come on, you knew that.)

I'm blessed that my basket is full of meaningful relationships, wonderful memories and acquired wisdom. My relationships and memories are personal and wouldn't mean much to you, but I can share from my cache of wisdom. It's the fruit of a life spent grappling with questions large and small.

Wisdom is distilled truth. It is absorbed through the skin—not the eyes or ears—and passed on through touch. It evaporates when hoarded and expands when shared. In that spirit, here's some of what I've learned so far:

- » And now abide information, knowledge and wisdom, but the greatest of these is wisdom.
- » Being alive means learning something new every day.
- » People are more important than possessions.
- » Relationships matter more than reputation.
- » Responsibility comes before reward.
- » Always thank the pilot. We only get where we want in life because of the skills of others.
- » Don't obsess over what people think about you; they don't.
- » Avoid books with numbers in the title; it's seldom that simple.
- » Change the world; spend time with your kids and grandkids.

Whatever the metaphors we use, the message is the same and

hasn't changed since the beginning: "For dust you are and to dust you will return" (Genesis 3:19).

○   ○   ○

"My body is filled with imperfections,
and one of them will get me."
—A. J. Jacobs

IN HOSPITAL

I check into Memorial Hospital on Tuesday morning, March 24, and cross the hall from the outpatient clinic to the inpatient side. The medical personnel are professional but not pushy. They treat me as a person, not a disease. (I'm sure it has nothing to do with me blogging everything that happens.)

This is what I appreciate most as a client, aka patient: The doctors and nurses come across as people first. Yes, they are highly trained specialists whose skills are saving my life, but we can talk and banter about other things, for example grandkids, the economy, good wine and bad doctor shows on TV. I even interviewed Dr. Dax and put the video on YouTube, along with other clips chronicling my battle with cancer.

In preparation for my transplant I must get a chemo cocktail of unpronounceable pharmaceuticals with the acronym RICE.

Rituximab is a monoclonal antibody wonder drug that works by targeting the CD20 antigen on B-cells. This drug was also the R in my RCHOP chemo.

Ifosfamide is an alkylating agent chemically related to the nitrogen mustards. Used for recurring cancers. Can cause hemorrhagic cystitis (bladder irritation).

Carboplatin is a cytotoxic alkylating agent that causes a dramatic decrease in the blood cell and platelet output of the bone marrow.

Etoposide (aka VP-16) is a type of topoisomerase inhibitor that blocks certain enzymes needed for cell division and DNA repair. And it may even kill cancer cells.

I have to have two rounds of RICE three weeks apart. It's more toxic than RCHOP, which is why I'm in the hospital. This is my first hospital stay since I had my tonsils out more than fifty years ago. Until recently, I've been extremely fortunate in the health department, having gone more than half a century without needing hospitalization.

How many people can say that!

Thursday evening I put on an impressive display of projectile vomiting. If this was a hotel I would've been asked to leave but they are forgiving about such indiscretions here. What it did get me was enough sleeping medicine to put me down for the entire night, a wonderful blessing.

I wake up at 5 a.m. on Friday with a full bladder to find myself neatly balanced on three pillows; one under my head, one under my butt and one under my heels. It is like sleeping on lily pads. I thank the nurse for arranging me as to minimize soakage in case of a breach in the levee but Nancy says she didn't do it.

I wonder who did?

Between Stays

I have raised four kids and written a dozen books but it is RICE chemo that finally gets me to pull my hair out by the roots. I stood over the wastebasket two weeks after I got out of the hospital and completely depilated my noodle. Now if someone tells me to go pluck myself I can say I already have. I don't want to go to tomorrow's Easter dinner bald as an egg but I'm shedding like a German Shorthair and Susan can't take me out in public. Plucking is easier than shaving and not too painful. My top is once more as smooth and shiny as a baby's bottom.

Only a person who's gone through chemo can know what it's like. I'm okay with losing my hair because I think I have a rather handsome head (it's the chemo talking) but I can understand how devastating it must be for women. My heart goes out to them.

My blood counts are low between chemo cycles, which brings me to a new word—and condition—for the week: "Thrombocytopenia." It means a low blood platelet count (PLT). Platelets (thrombocytes) are colorless cells made in the bone marrow, to the tune of about $1x10^{11}$ a day. They line the inside of blood vessels and play an important role in clotting, among other things. If you come up short due to disease or treatments like chemotherapy, you run the risk of increased bleeding with injury, excessive bruising and petechiae (red dots on the skin).

A normal platelet count is between one hundred fifty thousand to four hundred thousand cells/mm. I'm at about sixty-two thousand, which means I have to be careful. No playing with the neighbor's porcupine or rearranging my antique razor blade collection. No picking my nose with a nail file or flossing with piano wire. My main concern is that if my platelets don't rebound, it might put a kink in my stem cell transplant schedule. I do not want to get a penalty for delay of game.

It seems there is another bump on the road to transplant. My dentist found a problem that may require a root canal before the transplant. There's a dark spot beneath a crown that has to be cleared up lest it hold opportunistic bacteria that could be lethal once my immune system is destroyed.

Never a dull moment.

Tuesdays and Thursdays

Back in the hospital on Tuesday, April 15, for more RICE. For the first time since starting chemo I shed tears as I feel the initial flush of my eighth round. Perhaps it's a premonition that the day would be rough—it was—or the sleep short—that, too. But somehow I survive. I'm even able to go to the coffee shop a few times between infusions to write on my blog.

I've heard that RICE can be the hardest part of the stem cell transplant journey. If so, that means I'm cresting this mountain and starting downhill. Wait a minute; that doesn't sound good. How about, I'm coming to the easy part? Hmmm, stem cell harvesting, destruction of my immune system ...

Chemo is like riding a roller coaster; you have to learn when to relax and when to close your eyes and puke. And it's not a bad idea to let it scare the crap out of you because constipation only makes it worse.

I read the book *Tuesdays with Morrie* and found it enlightening, but Thursdays with Mikey are a nightmare. Lots going on and most of it is bad. It's the same as with my first round of RICE. It seems that surviving Thursdays is the key. That's the day the cart comes by in *Monty Python and the Holy Grail*:

CART MASTER:
Bring out your dead! [clang]
Bring out your dead! [cough cough ...] [clang]
Bring out your dead! [clang]
Bring out your dead! [clang]
Bring out your dead! Ninepence. [clang]
Bring out your dead! [clang]
CUSTOMER:
Here's one.
CART MASTER:
Ninepence.
DEAD PERSON:
I'm not dead!

CART MASTER:

What?

CUSTOMER:

Nothing. Here's your ninepence.

DEAD PERSON:

I'm not dead!

CART MASTER:

'Ere. He says he's not dead!

CUSTOMER:

Yes, he is.

DEAD PERSON:

I'm not!

CART MASTER:

He isn't?

CUSTOMER:

Well, he will be soon. He's very ill.

DEAD PERSON:

I'm getting better!

CUSTOMER:

No, you're not. You'll be stone dead in a moment.

CART MASTER:

Oh, I can't take him like that. It's against regulations.

DEAD PERSON:

I don't want to go on the cart!

CUSTOMER:

Oh, don't be such a baby.

CART MASTER:

I can't take him.

DEAD PERSON:

I feel fine!

CUSTOMER:

Well, do us a favor.

CART MASTER:
I can't.
CUSTOMER:
Well, can you hang around a couple of minutes? He won't be long.
CART MASTER:
No, I've got to go to the Robinsons'. They've lost nine today.
CUSTOMER:
Well, when's your next round?
CART MASTER:
Thursday.
DEAD PERSON:
I think I'll go for a walk.
CUSTOMER:
You're not fooling anyone, you know. Look. Isn't there something you can do?
DEAD PERSON: [singing]
I feel happy. I feel happy. [whop]
CUSTOMER:
Ah, thanks very much.
CART MASTER:
Not at all. See you on *Thursday*.

o   o   o

"Time rushes towards us with its hospital tray
of infinitely varied narcotics, even while it is preparing us
for its inevitably fatal operation."
—Tennessee Williams

DRUGGED OUT

W hen I get home from the hospital on April 20 it's a wonder I can sit up, much less stand. I don't know how to describe what chemo feels like. Instead I'll list all the drugs I've been given and you can deduce the consequences. Let your imagination go wild but have a bucket handy. Over the last eight months I've been repeatedly injected with, or ingested, a pharmacopeia from A to Z; either to kill the cancer or to minimize the side-effects of the "cure."

- » Ativan
- » Carboplatin
- » Clindamycin
- » Cyclophosphamide
- » Dexamethasone
- » Diphenhydramine
- » Doxorubicin
- » Etoposide
- » Filgrastim
- » Granisetron
- » Ifosfamide
- » Levaquin
- » Lunesta
- » Mesna
- » Ondansetron
- » Oxycodone
- » Prednisone
- » Prochlorperazine
- » Rituximab
- » Valtrex
- » Vincristine
- » Zolpidem

(This would be a killer list for the National Spelling Bee.)

The newest addition to my list of drugs to swallow—number twenty-three, but who's counting—is fluconazole (the generic of Diflucan), which my female readers will recognize as a leading treatment for yeast infections. The packaging boasts, "Just one oral tablet provides a full course of therapy sufficient to cure most vaginal yeast infections." Me? I'm on a fourteen-day regime. And yet I feel ill equipped to fully benefit.

So, my oncologist says to the pharmacist, "I bet we can get this guy to take anything!" (laughter)

"My oncologist is so concerned about my cancer spreading."
"How concerned is he?"
"He's got me protecting organs I don't have!" (rim shot)

Knock, knock.
Who's there?
Yeast.
Yeast who?
Yeast you won't have to worry about scratching yourself to death. (groan)

Actually, fluconazole is part of the "anti" phase of my transplant staging. I'm taking anti-fungal, anti-bacterial and anti-inflammatory meds to minimize problems and maximize the chances of a good harvest.

Drug of Choice
There is one drug that I enjoy along with 108 million other Americans—caffeine. I consider caffeine a vitamin, not a drug, and start most days with a cup of java. I usually have mine at Agia

Sophia's, my favorite coffee shop. The beans are freshly ground and brewed in a French press.

Coffee is one of the half dozen drinks that shaped civilization according to A History of the World in Six Glasses; the others being beer, wine, spirits, tea and Coca-Cola. Granted, coffee is an acquired taste. I learned to drink it at late-night elders' meetings. I used to think these marathon sessions were a measure of our dedication and commitment but later realized their length only reflected our incompetence.

Like some other things I enjoy, I used to feel guilty about drinking coffee because it was supposed to be bad for me. I limited myself to two or three cups a week although I was in restaurants almost daily for various meetings. But in time, greed overcame guilt. If I ordered hot chocolate or tea I got one cup whereas coffee came with free refills.

Knowledge has also put my mind at ease. To date there have been more than 19,000 studies regarding coffee's impact on health. The WebMD article, "Coffee: The New Health Food?" notes that,

> "Overall, the research shows that coffee is far more healthful than it is harmful," says Tomas DePaulis, PhD, research scientist at Vanderbilt University's Institute for Coffee Studies. ... "For most people, very little bad comes from drinking it, but a lot of good."
>
> Consider this: At least six studies indicate that people who drink coffee on a regular basis are up to 80% less likely to develop Parkinson's. ... Other research shows that compared to not drinking coffee, at least two cups daily can translate to a 25% reduced risk of colon cancer, an 80% drop in liver cirrhosis risk and nearly half the risk of gallstones.

Coffee consumption has also been shown to lower the risk of other maladies, from type 2 diabetes to Alzheimer's disease to cavities. It can increase cognitive performance and decrease the risk of suicide and is the leading contributor of antioxidants to the American diet.

I appreciate the medicinal benefits of coffee but that's not why I drink it. I use it as a way to signal my brain it's time to show up for work. I can't go as far as Balzac, who said, "As soon as coffee is in your stomach, there is a general commotion. Ideas begin to move … similes arise, the paper is covered with ink. … Coffee is your ally and writing ceases to be a struggle." He drank his coffee strong and black and produced about 100 novels and plays. I use cream and agave; maybe that's why my output is a fraction of his.

o   o   o

"Poisons and medicine are oftentimes the same substance
given with different intents."
—Peter Mere Latham

READ THIS, EAT THAT

hemotherapy isn't helping my diet because it messes with my appetite. I should turn my weight loss to my advantage by writing *The Lymphoma Diet Book*. It's the perfect plan for frustrated dieters: eat all you can, lounge around, no exercise required. True, it costs more than other weight-loss programs but it has better results. The name might need some work, though.

As long as we're talking imaginary books, here are some that might do well if written by the right people:

> » *Chemo Sabe: Famous People Who Beat Cancer* by Jay Silverheels, aka Tonto
> » *What's In It For Me? Using Cancer To Get Your Way* by Dennis Leary
> » *Born Under the Wrong Sign: Avoid Cancer by Changing Your Birthday* by John Edwards
> » *Procrastinator's Guide to Cancer* by Tom DeLay
> » *Cancer: Miracle Cure for Old Age* by Dr. Al Zheimer
> » *The Secret Life of Angiogenesis Inhibitors* by Sue Monk Kidd
> » *Outwitting Your Oncologist* by Scott (Deadbeat) Monteith (Based on the story of a patient whose oncologist gave him six months to live. When Scott couldn't pay his bill the doctor gave him another six months.)

Then there are the books on specific cancers:
- » *Tapeworms and Colon Cancer* by J. Wentworth Wigglebottom
- » *Simply Bursting: Relief from Bladder Cancer* by April Showers
- » *Licking Tongue Cancer* by Professor Grievous Maw
- » *Coming to Grips with Breast Cancer: A Hands-On Approach* by Dr. Joy Mounds

Anticancer

The best real book I've read on the subject is the number one selling cancer book in the world at this time, *Anticancer: A New Way of Life* by David Servan-Schreiber.

> After undergoing chemotherapy and surgery for brain cancer, Servan-Schreiber, a clinical professor of psychiatry at the University of Pittsburgh School of Medicine, asked his oncologist if any lifestyle changes would prevent a relapse; the answer was no. Certain this was wrong, Servan-Schreiber spent months researching a mass of scientific data on natural defenses against cancer.—*Publishers Weekly*

Dr. Servan-Schreiber's medical training and personal experience put him in a unique position to teach from the head *and* the heart. He doesn't disparage conventional medicine, as many alternative advocates do; nor does he dismiss the vast amount of data on the benefits of nutritional and lifestyle changes. He writes,

> Cancer lies dormant in all of us. Like all living organism, our bodies are making defective cells all the time. That's how tumors are born. But our bodies are also equipped with a number of mechanisms that detect and keep such cells in check. In the West, one person in four will die of cancer, but three of four will not. Their defense mechanism will hold out,

and they will die of other causes.

Cancer is more widespread today in the West and has been increasing since 1940. Hence, we must examine what has changed in our countries since World War II. Three major factors have drastically disrupted our environment over the last fifty years:

1. The addition of large quantities of highly refined sugar to our diet.
2. Changes in methods of farming and raising animals and, as a result, in our food.
3. Exposure to a large number of chemical products that didn't exist before 1904.

Studies on the activity of immune cells ... show that they are at their best when our diets are healthy, our environment is clean, and our physical activity involves the entire body (not just our brains and our hands). Immune cells are also sensitive to our emotions. Risk factors for cancer include:

» poor dietary habits: 30%
» smoking: 30%
» hereditary factors: 15%
» infection: 5%
» workplace exposure: 5%
» obesity and lack of exercise: 5%
» alcohol: 3%
» UV-ray exposure: 2%
» pollution: 2%
» other: 2%
» drugs: 1%

Natural Pharmaceuticals

Dr. Servan-Schreiber also offers some colorful dietary advice:

» Green tea [reduces] the growth of the new vessels needed for tumor growth and metastases. Drink two or three cups a day. Let steep for five to eight minutes.

» Turmeric [yellow powder used in curry] is the most powerful natural anti-inflammatory identified today. To be assimilated by the body, turmeric must be mixed with black pepper.

» Tomato sauce [which contains lycopene] leads to longer survival rates from prostate cancer in men who consume it in at least two meals a week. Tomatoes must be cooked in order to release their lycopene.

» Red wine [which contains resveratrol] acts on genes that are known to protect healthy cells against aging. It can also slow the three stages of cancer development. One glass a day with a meal.

» Dark chocolate [more than seventy percent cacao] contains a number of antioxidants whose molecules slow the growth of cancer cells. Mixing dairy products with chocolate cancels the beneficial effects of the molecules of cocoa. Avoid milk chocolate.

He recommends a book by fellow physicians Richard Beliveau and Denis Gingras that I've found very helpful. *Foods to Fight Cancer* points out:

The continuous presence of anti-angiogenic molecules as supplied through diet helps the body's natural defense mechanisms stop tumors at a harmless stage. ... The use of anticancer molecules present in food as a therapeutic weapon constitutes an essential method of maintaining these tumors at a latent stage and keeping them from progressing to an advanced stage of lethality.

The book details a cornucopia of cancer fighting foods, including:

- Brussels sprouts
- broccoli
- cauliflower
- cabbage
- garlic
- onions
- spinach
- watercress
- flax seeds
- tomato paste
- turmeric
- black pepper
- blueberries
- blackberries
- raspberries
- dried cranberries
- grapes
- dark chocolate (70% cacao)
- citrus fruit juice
- green tea
- red wine

Eating across this rainbow of colors and tastes is one way to help tip the scales of fate in your favor.

o   o   o

"Eat right, exercise regularly, die anyway."
—Author Unknown

RMBMT-07-C

O n the first two days in May I undergo seven medical tests and am conscious for all of them, meaning they aren't too stressful. The following Monday I have another bone marrow biopsy and on Tuesday I spend more than two hours in the dentist chair having a defective root canal redone. There's little pain thanks to nurse Novocain as Dr. Roth rooted (sic) around like a rigger looking for oil.

Keeping my jaw wide open for more than two hours was the main challenge. The old dentistry had been done with the equivalent of super glue and only the consummate skill of Dr. Roth keeps me from needing oral surgery to repair the problem. Getting a clean bill of health from a dentist is one of the many requirements before getting a bone marrow transplant.

Prepping, testing and doing all the paperwork for the transplant is a full-time job. Too bad it doesn't pay anything. The process is daunting, but mostly I feel humbled and a bit guilty at all this medical attention. More money is being spent on me than on whole Mexican villages dealing with the H1N1 flu!

I will start my pre-transplant prep at the Rocky Mountain Cancer Center (RMCC) in Denver on May 12. The packet of forms sent beforehand contains twenty-nine pages to review and sign. It's titled:

RMBMT-07-C
Treatment of Malignant Lymphoma with
High-Dose Carmustine, Etoposide, Cytarabine and
Cyclophosphamide (BEAC) or Melphalan (BEAM) followed by
Autologous Peripheral Progenitor Cell Rescue

The transplant process involves a dozen steps:
» initial evaluation
» induction chemotherapy
» pre-mobilization evaluation
» central venous catheter placement
» mobilization
» stem cell collection
» pre-transplant evaluation
» preparative regimen
» stem cell transplant
» post-chemotherapy
» engraftment
» recovery

I'm thankful I'll be in good hands. I've been very impressed with the people and procedures at RMCC. They do more than two hundred transplants a year and really know their stuff.

I will commute to Denver for the initial procedures. Once the heavy-duty stuff starts, Susan and I will move into the Staybridge Inn for several weeks. This is a welcome option given to autologous transplants patients instead of hospitalization.

While medical miracles are often worked in hospitals, they aren't places you want to stay if you can avoid them. According to a *Wall Street Journal* article, "How to Have a Safe Hospital Stay,"

Despite advances in medical care, hospital safety continues

to be a serious concern for patients. In 1999, the Institute of Medicine reported that an estimated 90,000 patients die from medical errors each year, a number that by some estimates has not changed and may even have increased. The threat of hospital infections is one key concern for patients; according to the Centers for Disease Control and Prevention healthcare-associated infections account for an estimated 1.7 million infections and 99,000 associated deaths each year. The non-profit Institute for Healthcare Improvement calculates that in total, nearly 15 million instances of medical harm occur in the U.S. each year—a rate of more than 40,000 per day.

Mobilization

On Friday, May 15, I start my mobilization chemotherapy at RMCC, my ninth round of chemo in the past ten months. This regimen stars Cytoxan and Etoposide, which I've had before. The former is an alkylating agent derived from mustard gas and the latter is a topoisomerase inhibitor. They are given as part of a three-day cycle to mobilize my stem cells for collection in a week or so. I'm put on a hydration pump around the clock and hooked to a second pump for Mesna. Cytoxan breaks down to produce acrolein, which is toxic to the bladder. Mesna binds to and inactivates it, preventing or reducing organ damage.

The mobilization chemo turns out to be pretty de-mobilizing. It's my worst yet as far as side effects. Next Friday, if my counts are up, I will begin stem cell collection, called apheresis. The harvested cells will be frozen and after a week of rest I'll start six days of "high-dose" chemo to kill off any remaining cancer cells. Unfortunately, it will also destroy my bone marrow and immune system and I will have to be engrafted with my stem cells to reboot my body.

Transplant day is known as Day 0. After that it usually takes two or three weeks for the stem cells to start producing new white blood cells, platelets and finally red blood cells. During this time the oncology staff will keep an eye on me while I do my best not to get infections or other complications. If all goes well, I'll be sent home somewhere between Day 20 and 28.

This should make for an unusual summer vacation. With a nod to David Letterman's Top Ten, I've come up with two lists of my own:

Ten Ways a Stem Cell Transplant Is Like a Luxury Vacation
1. You get six weeks away from home and work.
2. The logistics and financial arrangements are handled by specialists.
3. Accommodations are in a nice hotel in an upscale section of an international city.
4. A daily per diem is provided for travel and out-of-pocket expenses.
5. A live-in caregiver accompanies you whose sole purpose is to meet your every need.
6. Your health is monitored daily by some of the best doctors in the world.
7. You aren't allowed to do any housework, yard work, or labor of any kind.
8. There's abundant free time to read, relax, sleep, or sightsee, with special instructions to avoid crowds.
9. Eating and drinking as much as you can are strongly encouraged—*sans* alcohol—with the goal of gaining as much weight as possible.
10. A large corporation foots most of the bill; a good thing since this six-figure junket will probably be the most expensive excursion you'll ever take.

Ten Ways a Stem Cell Transplant Is *Not* Like a Luxury Vacation
1. You feel like the "morning after" without the "night before."

2. Alcohol is only for cleaning your catheter caps and port site.
3. Your "cocktails" aren't mixed by a sexy bartender but by a pharmacist in hazmat gear.
4. "Shooting up" means a Neupogen shot.
5. Forget sun bathing; fifteen minutes of direct sun can cause third-degree burns.
6. Risky activities aren't hang gliding and parasailing but flossing and nail clipping.
7. "Water sports" involve the bathroom, not the pool.
8. Your mouth feels like you've been sucking poison ivy Altoids.
9. "Sleeping in" refers to anything after 5:30 a.m.
10. The little blue pills you take are for sleeping, not sex (Lunesta, not Viagra).

o   o   o

"Try to relax and enjoy the crisis."
—Ashleigh Brilliant

APHERESIS TO INFUSION

On Tuesday and Wednesday, May 27 and 28, I park my keister in a blue recliner at Presbyterian St. Luke's Infusion Center for five hours of cell collection known as apheresis. The COBE Spectra machine next to me runs my blood through a centrifuge to separate its various components and skim off the peripheral stem cells—2.3 million on Tuesday and, hopefully, more today so I can go home tonight having been harvested of around five million cells.

By the time I'm done, my entire blood supply—five liters in my case—will have been out of my body and through the machine a dozen times. My collected stem cells will be frozen until I come back to Denver on June 7 to prep for my transplant. It takes ten hours to collect the cells but only fifteen minutes to put them back into my bone marrow. I thought they would have to be screened once more for cancer, but that isn't the case.

Stomatitis and Stigmata

After apheresis I get to go home for a few days before coming back to RMCC for my high-dose chemo to destroy any lingering cancer.

The chemotherapy is called "high-dose" because the doses received are from 5 to 10 times higher than the doses given during traditional chemotherapy. Such high doses of chemotherapy destroy cancer cells but also destroy other healthy cells in the body, which divide and reproduce rapidly, such as the cells that line the mouth, stomach, intestine and the bone marrow. … High-dose chemotherapy is the treatment used to destroy cancerous cells, while peripheral stem cell transplantation is necessary to "rescue" damaged bone marrow.

I continue to be plagued with the side effects of earlier chemo. One of the discomforts is mouth sores caused by stomatitis—an inflammation in the mouth—or oral mucositis—an irritation of the mucous lining of the mouth. The problem is that these linings aren't replaced as frequently as needed because chemo kills the body's fast-growing cells.

This is also why hair falls out, why nausea and diarrhea can occur and why some patients develop a tolerance for talk radio. Chemo can also affect the taste buds, of which we have about 10,000. It can temporarily rewire our perception of the five taste sensations: sweet, bitter, salty, sour and umami (whatever that means).

As with other side effects, mouth sores vary from person to person. They can show up a few days after treatment and take a few weeks to heal. They are temporary, except when you've had as much chemo as I have; then they just become part of life. Thankfully mine aren't severe.

These are the major means of minimizing mouth maladies:

» avoid spicy, sour, coarse, or crunchy foods;
» brush frequently with a soft brush;
» rinse regularly with a baking soda-salt solution to discourage the growth of bacteria;
» use topical analgesics like lidocaine or xylocaine and coating agents such as kaopectate or sucralfate.

When I got sores with my first chemo, I tried a prescription called Magic Mouthwash. The only thing "magic" was the price—sixty dollars for fourteen ounces. Since then I've reverted to what my grandma used for good oral hygiene: baking soda. And she lived to be 104.

I am sitting at my computer one night and suddenly realize my arm is bleeding. The same thing has happened twice before in the last few days. Had the blood been on my hands, I could have claimed stigmata, of which there have been more than five hundred recorded cases; the most famous involving St. Francis of Assisi. But it's actually a secular condition known as petechiae.

Petechiae are tiny subcutaneous dots formed by blood seeping from the capillaries. They are caused by thrombocytopenia—a low platelet count. After two days of stem cell collection, my platelet count had dropped to 15,000, hence the spontaneous bleeding. Any lower and I would have had to have an infusion before coming home.

Not to worry. Since my bone marrow turns out about 1×10^{11} new platelets daily I should be in the pink—a figure of speech since platelets are colorless—by Monday.

Knockout Round

The high-dose regime starts on Monday June 8, and lasts for six days. The weekend before, Susan and I move into the Staybridge Inn where RMCC has reserved a block of rooms for transplant patients. We make arrangements with the hotel to remove the couch so we can bring our own recliners. We might as well be comfortable since we'll be here for several weeks. There's a Super Target across the street and a nice walking trail behind the hotel. Shotgun Willie's is down the block, but visiting a gentleman's club isn't on our itinerary.

Here's my menu for the week:

Drinks and appetizers:
» Saline solution
» Scopalomine anti-nausea patch
» Dexamethasone

Main courses:
» Carmustine
» Cytarabine
» Etoposide
» Melphalan

Side (effect) dishes:
» Compazine
» Kytril
» Lansoprazole
» Lorazepam
» Temazepam

Dessert (next week):
» Acyclovir
» Diflucan
» Levaquin

My treatment ends on Saturday with a final bag of Melphalan and an electrolyte chaser. Sunday is a rest day and I'll get my stem cells back on Monday, June 15, aka Day 0. The chemo effects will reach their worst about two weeks later. That's also about how long it will take for my stem cells to engraft in my bone marrow and start making new blood products. I'll have to be very careful during this time but at least I'll be in the home stretch.

Day 0: Infusion

Monday, June 15: The 4.7 million cells collected a few weeks ago are put back in today. This infusion is the "rescue" part of the operation. It takes only fifteen minutes. This is called engraftment. I will be monitored daily during the following weeks while my blood, bone marrow and immune system regenerate.

Infusion is a painless but stinky business. Short-term side effects include bad breath and rancid body odor caused by the DMSO solution used to keep the frozen stem cells from crystallizing. Poor Susan. She has to endure the stench at close quarters.

Starting tomorrow I have to go to the clinic every morning for blood tests and treatment according to my daily deficiencies. I'll be on anti-everything drugs and will get transfusions as needed because

> Until engraftment is complete, a transplant recipient is susceptible to infection, anemia, and bleeding caused by low blood cell counts. Therefore, special precautions are necessary during recovery. Patients may be given red blood cell and platelet transfusions during the recovery period to help prevent anemia and bleeding. … On the average, it takes about 2 to 3 months to recover normal physical performance after an autologous procedure. However, it can take as long as a year for a patient to get back to his or her normal routine (http://www.multiplemyeloma.org/treatmens/3.03.php).

After all this medically inflicted suffering, is there a chance the cancer will return? Yes, but there are two characteristics of non-

Hodgkin lymphoma that are in my favor:

» NHL is a cancer of the white blood cells circulating in the lymphatic system. Very few cancerous cells are actually in the blood, which is where the stem cells are harvested.

» Apheresis (cell collection) harvests only stem cells, not white blood cells.

However, the process is far from perfect and some blood products are inadvertently collected along with the stem cells. This means there's a risk of getting the cancer back. But it's less risky than doing nothing at all. So I choose to focus on one day at a time. That's all any of us has, whether we think we are in good health or are struggling for survival.

o   o   o

"Now listen, you who say,
'Today or tomorrow we will go to this or that city,
spend a year there, carry on business and make money.'
Why, you do not even know what will happen tomorrow.
What is your life? You are a mist that appears for a little while
and then vanishes. Instead, you ought to say,
'If it is the Lord's will, we will live and do this or that.'"
—James 4:13-15

AFTERMATH

P ainful as it has been, my transplant has gone well thus far. A bone marrow transplant is not something you want on your bucket list. It's not an easy medical procedure to endure; it's only tolerable because in most cases the alternative is death. Compared to what others have faced, I consider myself a novice at suffering. Fellow writer, blogger and veteran cancer fighter Ronni Gordon, (www.runnerwrites.blogspot.com) has survived four transplants.

I got really sick (105-degree fevers) after my induction in 2003. I had an auto and was good for three and a half years. I thought I was done with it, but then I relapsed. I didn't get too sick with the next two ... I rejected the first graft after six months. They don't know why. They didn't think it was the donor so they gave me the same donor a second time.

That time at six months the leukemia snuck back in despite the donor and I relapsed. This time they gave me a double dose of some chemo that hopefully got rid of the leukemia for good, plus a transplant from a different donor (Jan. 31). I'm 100 percent engrafted, but the chemo nearly did me in ... kidney failure, infections, fevers, coma, the works. So here I sit trying to stay positive. It's not always easy but as we all know, that's what we have to do.

Why fight so hard and endure so much? Because life is precious. Not as a single spark but as a shared experience with family, friends and others. I'm looking forward to playing with my grandkids and to growing old with Susan. I want to do more laughing around the table with my kids, to have more philosophical discussions over coffee with my buddies and to convert as many strangers as I can into friends.

These are my reasons to do whatever it takes to stay alive.

In Praise of Pus

My desire may be to spend time with others but my reality currently revolves around a pole. Not the kind they have down the block at Shotgun Willie's, or the professional model they use at the clinic, but my own personal IV pole. I'm tethered to it five times a day and shot in the chest with antibiotics by my wife-nurse. I'm not complaining because it seems to be curing my infection.

When we see pus, it's a thick, usually yellowish-white ooze of degenerating white blood cells, tissue debris, protein, skin cells and dead or dying microorganisms. Pus consists of large numbers of white cells called polymorphonuclear cells that rush to a specific area of the body in response to infection. These cells engulf and kill harmful bacteria and also enlarge nearby blood vessels to bring more white cells to the scene of the crime, hence the inflammation.

In my current condition, when the sores on my hand and leg—one the size of a quarter and the other as big as a silver dollar—call 911, no one answers. Talk about a budget shortfall! My body is bankrupt and there are no emergency services available. However, I'm getting outside help in the form of three or four more drugs that Susan has to give me several times daily. These are triage measures; I should be making my own pus again by next week. How's that for a specific life goal: Make pus?

My engraftment is starting to take hold. My white count has climbed above 1 k/mcL; the average person's is closer to 10 on a good day. My platelets are at 25 k/mcL; the norm is between 150 and 400. But at least I've left Ground Zero!

I've been having night sweats for the past week. It starts with a teeth-chattering flood and slows to a pervasive drizzle. (Thankfully no urine is involved.) It's a good thing the hotel has a king-size bed as I can roll from damp to dry terrain for most of the night. And a great thing they have housekeeping to deal with the soggy aftermath. My tipping has gone way up. Sleep hyperhidrosis is the medical term for night sweats. Of its most common causes I can rule out:

» menopause and hormone disorders
» early sign of lymphoma
» reaction to medications
» hypoglycemia
» HIV
» neurologic conditions
» sleeping without an air conditioner

The probable cause, in descending order of likelihood:

» side effect of engraftment
» lingering infection
» sign of some lung damage done by the BCNU chemo

Prednisone has been added to my daily medications for the nightly perspiration and for a persistent cough, which could also indicate lung problems.

T+16
I've taken to adding "T+ #" to my signature, which stands for the number of days post-transplant. July 1 is T+16. I got off one drug

Monday and two more yesterday. My white counts and platelets are slowly climbing (5.3 and 92 respectively), which means my old-new stem cells are engrafted and doing their amazing work.

Engraftment feels like getting the flu—body aches, weight loss (I'm at 152 pounds), low-grade fever, night sweats—but it's all for a good cause. I keep telling myself feeling bad is part of getting better. If there are no setbacks, I'll have my exit interview and get my Hickman line out next Monday. I can go home on Tuesday, with a follow-up appointment a week later. I'll be on one set of restrictions till the end of July and another till the middle of September. Then it's just a matter of how quickly I recover my health and energy.

The transplant has been a success. It remains to be seen if the cancer will return, which happens in about forty percent of cases. I'm not concerned about that right now; I'm just taking one grace-day at a time.

o   o   o

"As I see it, there's a decision we all have to make,
and it seems perfectly captured in the
Winnie-the-Pooh characters created by A. A. Milne.
Each of us must decide: Am I a fun-loving Tigger
or am I a sad-sack Eeyore? Pick a camp."
—Randy Pausch

HOME AGAIN

I have my exit interview and Hickman line taken out on Monday, July 6. Another mountain in my sojourn on planet Earth has been summited; however, life is a serrated range, not a single peak. The best we can do is keep moving, enjoy the scenery, aim for the passes, avoid wildlife that weighs more than us and never travel alone. After a few more tests I get to come home.

It's great to be back in Colorado Springs and to sleep in my own bed. The transplant was a success. My bone marrow was destroyed and my clean stem cells engrafted. They are now busy producing white blood cells and platelets but it will be a while before I start growing red blood cells, hence the fatigue.

I've been rebooted; it remains to be seen if there is any cancer left in the system. I'll get my first post-transplant scan in September. The only lingering cloud is some probable lung damage caused by the BCNU chemo. The treatment for this is ten weeks of Prednisone, with the potential side effects of insomnia, cataracts and skin cancer.

Tour de Vie

I've been following the *Tour de France*, primarily because of the return to the epic race of Lance Armstrong, seven-time winner and fellow cancer survivor. This ninety-sixth Tour is comprised of twenty-one stages over twenty-three days and covers about twenty-two thousand miles. It's like pedaling north-to-south across the United States balanced on the spine of a Harry Potter book.

The longest stage is 139 miles and eight stages are in the mountains. The best time at the end of each day earns the *Maillot Jaune* or Yellow Jersey.

Women have never been allowed in the Tour because its founder, Henri Desgrange, felt the grueling physical demands were too much for female cyclists. There is a women's Tour held in August called the *Grande Boucle Feminine Internationale* that's about one-third as long.

Many people don't realize that although there is an individual winner, the Tour is a team sport. Each team starts with nine riders who work together doing whatever it takes to get their man on the winner's podium in Paris. There are twenty teams in this year's Tour.

Armstrong rides for team Astana, but not in the lead role. After teammate Alberto Contador decisively won the mountainous fifteenth stage, Armstrong said, "As far as I'm concerned, I'm happy to be a *domestique* (support rider). ... This is a team sport. I think now is the time for me to put my chances aside and focus on the team."

Domestiques haul water and food from team cars, protect their teammates from the opposing teams and help fix mechanical problems, including giving up their wheels or whole bikes if needed. Cyclist and writer Roger St Pierre explains,

> It is team tactics which so often win or lose races—and the lieutenants and the dog soldiers who expend their energy blocking chasing moves when they have riders up the road in a position to win. It is they who ride out into the wind so their aces can get an easier ride tucked inside their wheel. Rare indeed is the major victory that cannot be credited in large part to the groundwork laid by the *domestiques*.

Life is a lot like the Tour: it burns huge amounts of calories; unfurls in various stages; spans a variegated terrain; and requires team effort to succeed. If you had to name your Team, the one group with which you most identify, would it be family, friends, schoolmates, neighbors, work associates, church members or ministry partners? When was the last time you served them as a *domestique*? If you can't recall, put this book down and go provide some tactical support for a teammate.

○   ○   ○

"Make a list of the people who have shaped your life,
and try to figure out why."
—Phillip Yancey

NOT DEAD AT FIFTY-SIX

Having just celebrated my fifty-seventh birthday on July 29, I'm so thankful not to have joined the likes of Abraham Lincoln, Beethoven and Hitler, who all died at age fifty-six. A year ago I was diagnosed with non-Hodgkin lymphoma, which was a downer at my last birthday party. I didn't know what lay ahead then. Probably a good thing. During the past year I've undergone

» multiple scans, biopsies, tests and procedures;
» four port surgeries;
» six rounds of RCHOP chemo;
» two rounds of RICE chemo, requiring hospitalization;
» mobilization and high-dose chemotherapies;
» bone marrow transplant.

Along with bags of weapons-grade chemicals whose names I can't pronounce, I've been injected with or ingested a plethora of

» anti-inflammatory meds;
» anti-bacterial meds;
» anti-fungal meds;
» anti-nausea meds;
» sleeping pills;
» steroids.

Despite the best medical care, I've had my share of
  » insomnia;
  » fatigue;
  » nausea;
  » vomiting;
  » night sweats;
  » infections;
  » fevers.

All these inconveniences are put into perspective by a single reality—*Life!* I'm still here, by the grace of God, and feeling stronger every day.

I'm two months post stem cell transplant and doing well, especially compared to others whose stories I've read. I have so much to be thankful for. I'm sleeping without the aid of pills for the first time in a year. My hair is growing; it looks and feels like dryer lint. I'm exercising and running again. True, I'm slower than a lobbying reform bill in Congress but at least I'm moving. I've regained half the weight I lost over the course of chemo.

I do have ongoing areas of concern though. I still take more than thirty pills a week but the numbers will shrink with time. My cholesterol and triglycerides are still high and I can't figure out why. I may wind up on medication for this—more pills. Nothing new on the job front; this is the most discouraging part of life these days.

Then there's The Shadow.

Cancer casts a long shadow. Just because the transplant was successful doesn't mean my cancer is gone. Around sixty percent of people with non-Hodgkin lymphoma who get a transplant are alive five years later. Much better odds than if you do nothing; still, no slam-dunk. Then there are the secondary cancers to which the alkylating agents in my chemotherapy make me more susceptible, but let's not go there now.

Spandrels

A spandrel is the somewhat triangular space between two arches or between an arch and a rectangular enclosure. It is created incidentally by the juxtaposition of more important components. I'm using the term metaphorically to refer to the "accidental" spaces created by the main story arches in our lives and to what we fill those spaces with—like this book, which occupies a space inadvertently formed by two realities that give structure to who I am.

Arch One: I am a writer. What makes someone a writer? At its simplest, he or she writes. It's a compulsion that has to be expressed daily. In my case I've kept a journal for more than forty years. I've worked on magazines and websites and published a dozen books so far. I haven't sold anything to a publisher since 2004. Still, I keep writing. I've done six more children's books that no one is interested in and I've got ideas for a few adult books but no way to get them to an audience.

Arch Two: I have cancer. Cancer is a reality I've lived with for the past fifteen months (at this point) and despite a successful stem cell transplant its pall hangs over the future. I've read and researched cancer in general and non-Hodgkin lymphoma in particular. I've experienced firsthand much of what I've studied.

Based on the number of hits and reader comments on my blog, I believe many have been helped by my candid musings on things physical and spiritual. I've developed mutually beneficial relationships based on common questions and shared suffering. My blog may wind up having more impact than anything else I've written. I wouldn't have guessed—or chosen—this in the past but now it's something I wouldn't have missed.

I'm sure you have a spandrel or two in your life—some empty spaces between arches, unplanned and unused. Don't let them go to waste. Be proactive and creative. Try something new. Take a few risks. Improvise. Invent. When our cathedrals are complete I suspect the incidental will turn out to be important and the mundane may be spotlighted as the showcase of the divine.

○   ○   ○

"Life is like sailing.
You can use any wind to go in any direction."
—Robert Brault

PART III
ACCIDENT AND SURGERIES

AUGUST 2009 – DECEMBER 2010

"Pain is greedy, boorish, meanly debilitating.
It is cruel and calamitous and often constant, and, as its Latin
root *poena* implies, it is the corporal punishment each of us
ultimately suffers for being alive."
—Russell Martin

TOUGH BREAK

I was on my way to the Memorial clinic to see my oncologist on Tuesday, August 25, when a car pulled in front of me and introduced me to my airbag. I made the rest of the trip in an ambulance, my first time in said conveyance.

I vividly remember the crash and subsequent events: the cacophony of crunching metal, the stringent smell of a deflated airbag, the soft grass beneath my head as I lay on the ground and the wail of the approaching siren. I wince whenever I see a car crash in the movies or on TV and smirk when the people hop out and run off. You may be shocked to learn that's not how it is.

Here are the painful details.

The street I was on had just narrowed to one lane when a dark-colored sedan pulled out of a side street. I slammed on the brakes but there was no time to stop. I ended up ramming into the passenger-side door. My airbag deployed so fast that all I saw was a limp white balloon draped over the steering wheel.

My car did a 180 and wound up hopping the curb. I had a stabbing pain in my lower back so I unbuckled my belt and rolled out onto the grass. That's where the firemen found me a few minutes later. They applied a neck brace, strapped me on a body board and slid me into an ambulance. The driver of the other car was inside—a lady I guessed to be in her late sixties. She had a cut on her forehead but otherwise seemed okay. She was concerned about me and I can only imagine how she felt.

We ended up at the same hospital but I never saw her after that and was discouraged from making any contact until the insurance had been sorted out. Subsequently she was charged with careless driving, as is standard for anyone causing an accident resulting in serious injury. But as I told the DA later when asked if I wanted to say anything at her trial, there was no malice aforethought and I bear the lady no ill will. Accidents happen.

When I got to the ER I was X-rayed and CAT-scanned while still strapped to the board. Turns out I had a broken back—compression fractures of vertebras T2 and L5—a fractured sternum and bruised ribs (also a torn rotator cuff and a broken bone in my foot that I didn't realize until later). I had some spots on my lung that could have been contusions or else damage from the chemo I'd recently undergone. No surgery was required, just lots of time for the body to heal.

Coincidentally, Susan was on her way to work a few minutes after the accident and saw the smashed cars. She stopped when she realized one of them was mine. It didn't help her nerves that she found my hat lying in the road. The policeman told her I was fine and had been taken to the hospital with a cut on my forehead. He evidently got the two victims mixed up. Susan showed up at the ER before I could call her. My daughter Julie arrived a short time later and the rest of the family came as they heard the news.

I spent the next three days in the hospital being examined by various specialists. I was issued a body brace to be worn for the next few months whenever I'm not in bed. The hard plastic restraint reached from my collarbone to my hips. Front and back are held together with Velcro straps.

I wouldn't have survived the next several weeks if the brace hadn't been removable. I asked my family to come up with a name to go along with my new superhero outfit. My sister Kathy ended up suggesting the winner a few days later—Captain Crunch.

Tears and Trials

I got to go home on Friday and had real trouble getting into the car for the trip. The six-mile journey was a nightmare and I was in tears by the time we pulled into the garage. I managed to get upstairs and into bed with a lot of help. Susan had to lay me down, which was hard on her own back condition. Even with the pain pills I couldn't get comfortable. My low back was seized up and my sternum throbbed when I breathe. It was impossible to sleep.

Taking a shower in the body brace was awkward. Afterwards, Susan had to put me on the bed and wash my back. Then the contraption was clamped tight around me, usually for fifteen-plus hours a day. It was almost more painful than my injuries. I had trouble concentrating and I couldn't sit at my computer for long.

They say to take it easy for at least the first year after a stem cell transplant while your body recuperates. The accident occurred less than two months after I got home. It's a tough break, but it could have been worse. I was just getting back into running and now I could barely get around. My right foot hurt. When I got it X-rayed I learned why. Turns out I had a broken bone that didn't register on my pain radar while I was immobile. I had little appetite and when I did eat I got indigestion because of the tightness of the brace. Some nights I took it off early and sat very still in my chair watching TV, waiting for ten o'clock so I can take my sleeping pill.

o o o

"Without TV, it is hard to know
when one day ends and another begins."
—Homer Simpson

GETTING PHYSICAL

The human body is one complicated marvel of physical machinery. It doesn't help that I'm recovering from a full-system reboot, aka stem cell transplant, or that my injuries are incompatible. I'm in a body brace for my back but a fractured sternum usually isn't wrapped or placed in any type of restraint because the best healing occurs when you're able to breathe and move regularly rather than in a restricted manner.

A physical therapist comes by the house twice a week in September since I can't go anywhere yet. Kelly is helping my body deal with the trauma of the crash and get on with the healing process.

My lower back is tight and the pain is a constant ache punctuated by flashes of brilliance when I move the wrong way. My sternum is tender and doesn't hurt unless I annoy it; and then the pain is acute. There's a tightness between my shoulder blades and I can't lie on my left side because of my ribs. I'm by myself most of the day and can't do much. Susan helped me put on my shoes on Saturday and I walked down to the mailbox.

Here's my list of normal activities in increasing order of painfulness, from "no sweat" to "just shoot me":

» sit
» stand

» walk
» hug
» yawn
» laugh
» get in and out of bed
» isometric exercises
» burp
» hiccup
» cough
» sneeze

My daily life has changed dramatically; I have to use some new tools to get by:
» long-handle back scrubber (hospital issue)
» Featherlite Reacher, aka The Grabber (wish I'd invented this)
» breath tester (for checking lung capacity)
» sock sleeve (easy to operate)

Here's what the hospital charged for some of this take-home gear:
» back scrubber - $24.50
» Featherlite Reacher - $116.25
» breath tester - $107.50
» sock sleeve - $107.50

And the off-the-shelf body brace? Would you believe $2,457! Still, I'm thankful for the things I *don't* need:
» halo
» wheelchair
» breathing tube
» oxygen tank
» coffin

What's Up, Doc?

I was scheduled to be in Denver on Tuesday, September 8, for the first follow-up visit with Dr. Brunvand, my transplant doctor, but the accident has put a real kink in my recovery program. Instead, I see the trauma surgeon who treated me after my accident. There's nothing more he can do, so he signs off on my case. Tomorrow I see Dr. Do, the orthopedic surgeon on duty in the ER when I was brought in. She should be able to give me a better idea of my long-term prognosis and treatment.

Also on Wednesday I finally make it to the oncology appointment I was headed to on the day of the crash. All Dr. Dax can do is check my blood. There's no way to tell what's happening on the cancer front without a PET scan and I can't get one until my innards heal.

Two weeks later I see yet another kind of doctor; a physical injury physician who will be in charge of my recovery treatment. Dr. Leppard is encouraged that I don't have more pain and will start working with me more aggressively once I get out of this brace. I'm going to call Dr. Do to see if I can get time off my incarceration for good behavior. For now, I'm supposed to walk as much as possible. I can also exercise with light weights. I hope this will give me more energy as I run out of gas by the afternoon and have trouble getting anything done that involves concentration or creativity.

I'm not done with new physicians yet. On Tuesday, September 22, I go to a new GP (General Practitioner). Dr. Jewell will monitor my overall health and it takes him almost an hour to sort through the medical baggage I come with.

I've seem more docs in the past year than a Chinese freighter. I'm thankful for their skill and helpfulness but could do with a little less face time. Then there's the paperwork associated with the accident, which is a full-time job. It involves collecting and coordinating information from:

» four doctors and counting

» three insurance companies
» one hospital
» one physical therapist
» one attorney

All this is in addition to managing the ongoing logistics of my cancer, which involves a plethora of physicians, clinics, hospitals, laboratories, offices and other institutions, plus enough forms and reports to fill a file drawer. I need a separate drawer for my accident paperwork as I can't mix the two.

My workday is much shorter now; so is my attention span. The body brace hurts about as much as the condition it is correcting. It morphs into a torture device by the end of the day. Thankfully I don't have to sleep in it. I'm not one to whine and complain, so we'll just call this "sharing."

o   o   o

Goodnight Prayer
Now I lay me down to sleep;
I pray the Lord my back to keep.
For I am weak without my brace,
and needful of unmoving grace.

My sternum and my spine agree,
there's very little room for me
to wander from the narrow way;
I may not stir, I must not stray.

For if I twist or turn or strain,
this causes me no little pain,

and I give voice to yelps and groans,
the protest of my fractured bones.

Once down I can't get up to pee;
a handheld urinal, that's the key.
It's not a problem in the dark;
so long as I don't miss the mark.

As night by night my health improves;
this makes it easier to snooze.
To be at peace, this is God's will;
as meted out by sleeping pill.

In calmness I recline and rest,
no turtle shell on back or breast.
Despite the hurt, it's not that grim,
for Susan's here to tuck me in.
—Mike Hamel

PAIN SCALE

Everyone experiences pain but in such an individualistic and indescribable way. We all have our own vocabularies for the difficulties that afflict us. We have mechanical devices to evaluate everything from bone density (X-ray), to organ function (MRI), to cell formation (PET scan), but we have nothing to quantify pain. Like beauty, it is in the eye of the individual. The nouns may be the same—cancer, surgery, shoulder, stomach—but the adjectives that describe our discomforts are intimately ours.

The language of pain is so subjective that the medical community has to objectify it somehow. They've come up with scales of various sorts, the two most popular being the Visual Analog Scale (VAS) and the Face Pain Scale. Both use numbers from one to ten to categorize pain. This helps them do science but it does little to communicate the pathos of pain. After all, what does a "6" feel like to you? To me?

Several times in the last few months I've been asked to "choose a number from one to ten that describes your pain." The higher the number, the stronger the drugs administered. These simple subjective scales are used because there is no machine to measure pain. Some people resist pain and concede little to its onslaught.

Others are overwhelmed by the least discomfort. Neither approach is right or wrong; it just is.

The human body is hardwired for pain with millions of specialized nerves that monitor heat, cold, pressure and a myriad of other sensations. They make us instantly aware of damaging influences and motivate us toward healthy behavior, in my case like not crashing into other cars. Conversely, there's not a single nerve in the body expressly designed for registering pleasure. Feelings of well being, happiness and joy are controlled by neurotransmitters in the brain. To use a computer analogy, pain is a matter of hardware while pleasure is a matter of software.

Pain involves the body—including the brain—but it's the mind that determines suffering. The First Noble Truth of Buddhism says that, "Pain in life is inevitable, but suffering is not. Pain is what the world does to you; suffering is what you do to yourself. Pain is inevitable, suffering is optional."

I agree with the distinction but not the conclusion, which is overly optimistic. Pain is an inescapable part of existence and we usually don't have a choice as to its timing or intensity. How much we suffer from it is something we can address but not eliminate.

How different life would be without pain and suffering! Eternal banishment of these hydra-headed beasts after the final indignity of death is the hope to which we cling.

In the meantime, take a number.

Chronic Conditions

A "chronic" ailment is a persistent and lasting condition (from three months to life). To my chronic disease—cancer—I've added a chronic injury—crushed disc. The National Institute of Neurological Disorders and Stroke reports that "back pain is the second most common neurological ailment in the United States—only headache is more common. Americans spend at least $50 billion a year on low back pain."

According to the study, *Chronic Care in America: A 21st Century Challenge*, "Nearly one in two Americans has a chronic medical condition of one kind or another. However, most of these people are not actually disabled, as their medical conditions do not impair normal activities. ... The most common chronic conditions are high blood pressure, arthritis, respiratory diseases like emphysema and high cholesterol."

Chronic ailments make us painfully aware of our bodies. They are indeed "fearfully and wonderfully made," even when they malfunction. What should astound us daily is how much goes *right* with such complex mechanisms!

We have only to go skin deep to become overwhelmed. The epidermis is our largest organ, covering an average area of twenty-five square feet and containing forty-five miles of nerves. Every square inch is nourished by twenty feet of blood vessels and populated with thirty-two million bacteria. We shed and regrow about twenty-four ounces of skin a year, which means a new set of clothes for the emperor once every twenty-seven days and almost a thousand different outfits in a lifetime.

The skin conceals

» more than two hundred bones—a quarter of which are in our feet;

» more than six hundred muscles—about forty percent of our weight;

» sixty thousand miles of blood vessels that are kept full by a heart that beats an average of 2.5 billion times between the cradle and the grave.

Running the show is the brain, an aquatic organ comprised

of eighty percent water, leaving about seven ounces of solid tissue to do all the work. This spongy mass accounts for two percent of our weight yet consumes twenty percent of our intake of calories and oxygen.

But far and away the most interesting aspect of the body is that it interfaces with the soul, aka person, mind, self, spirit. It is the essence of who we are but whose essence we cannot locate or measure. It is what gives meaning to the body. It endows this life with purpose and the next with hope.

○　○　○

"You don't have a soul.
You are a Soul.
You have a body."
—C. S. Lewis

TYPICAL WEEKS

I get my latest PET scan on Tuesday, September 29. It should have been done a month ago but my auto accident postponed everything. It's the first scan I've had since my stem cell transplant in June and it will reveal what's happening on the cancer front.

I've mentioned PET scans earlier but here are a few more details as to how Positron Emission Tomography works. The "scanee" is injected with a tracer isotope, which collects in high glucose-using cells such as the brain, the liver and rapidly growing tumors. After about an hour the patient is put into an imaging scanner that records the energy given off by the isotope in high definition 3-D pictures that can be manipulated and studied from any angle.

A PET scan differs from a CT (computed tomography) scan or an MRI (magnetic resonance imaging) in that it reveals changes on the cellular level whereas a CT or MRI detects changes in the structure of organs or tissues. The apparatus itself is actually two massive doughnuts with a sliding table through the center. The first machine is a CT scanner and the second a PET scanner. The two technologies are combined in what's called co-registration. This fusion gives radiologists both anatomic (structural) and metabolic (biochemical) information simultaneously.

PET scans are especially useful for diagnosing, staging and

monitoring treatment of cancers, particularly lymphomas. That's why I've had several.

Good thing they're painless.

I get three reports the week of October 6, two of them good.

Dr. Dax gives me my PET scan results. There are no signs of cancerous activity in my lymph nodes! The X-rays done at the time of my accident showed some lesions in my right lung but these have shrunk since then so they're probably related to the accident or an infection and not cancer.

Dr. Do takes another set of X-rays and reports that my back is healing fine. I can shed my body brace, which is a great relief. I can also resume driving but not running. It's been more than six weeks since I've been behind the wheel and I'm looking forward to being more mobile.

Dr. Jewell tells me the results of my bone density scan: I have osteopenia, the precursor to osteoporosis. My mom had osteoporosis, which may be where I got it. Chemotherapy can also cause osteoporosis. The bottom line is that my bones fracture more easily. If my car accident had been three or four years earlier my injuries might not have been as severe.

Monday through Friday

Here's a typical week in the life of a cancer survivor/accident victim:

Monday, October 19: I take a pulmonary test to see if I have any lung damage from the high-dose chemo this summer. Probably not, since the results are similar to the test I had in May. (And very similar to a test I had in 1982.)

Tuesday: It's been eight weeks since the crash and I'm getting a bit more mobile each day. Still not supposed to run, work out my abs, or use dumbbells over five pounds.

Wednesday: I start physical therapy and I hope it will loosen the kinks and get rid of the soreness. I'd like to be able to turn my head freely in both directions—a useful skill now that I'm driving again.

Thursday: I pick up the new suit I bought for my trip to Washington, DC, next week to participate in a lawsuit against the US government.

Friday: I return to the Rocky Mountain Cancer Center for my first post-transplant exam—two months late because of my accident. Dr. Brunvand confirms that my lung lesions have improved, which means they were not caused by the high-dose chemo.

This week I also received my monthly social security disability check. I applied for disability after being diagnosed with cancer. Since non-Hodgkin lymphoma is on their list of terminal diseases I was approved with no hassle. If you have cancer, you may qualify to get some of the money back you've been paying into the system all these years. The place to check is the Disability page of the Social Security Administration's Web site.

President Ronald Reagan once famously said the nine most terrifying words in the English language are, "I'm from the government and I'm here to help." But in my case the government's been a big help. They've sent me unemployment checks when I couldn't work and disability payments when I got sick. Despite all the excesses and inequities, the system does work for a lot of Americans, and I, for one, deeply appreciate it.

Doctor visits aside, I spend a lot of time by myself. Writing is a lonely profession, especially when you don't have collaborative projects to work on. Having a home office doesn't help. And then there's injury and illness, which can lead to bouts of isolation.

Isolation isn't good for the soul. We are born with the innate need to connect with others, as is well documented in the book, *Hooked*, by Joe S. McIlhaney Jr., MD and Freda McKissic Bush, MD. "Connectedness for the average, healthy person is a part of who we are and how we function. It is wired into our brains when we are still in our mother's womb. This connectedness is passed on by our genes and is necessary for us to survive and thrive as healthy, capable persons."

I miss being able to go to Sophia's in the morning. I miss meeting friends and potential clients for coffee or Happy Hour. I miss people.

According to *Kinky Friedman's Guide to Texas Etiquette*, "You can pick your friends and you can pick your nose, but you can't wipe your friends off on your saddle." I'm thankful for true friends who haven't wiped me off in spite of my physical infirmities and spiritual wanderings. Through the years I've enjoyed camaraderie with small groups of men who tolerate and even encourage me. They listen to my babblings, wince at my heresies and laugh at my warped sense of humor, being somewhat warped themselves.

Next to family, true friends are the most cherished gifts I've been given in life.

o   o   o

"Without friends no one would choose to go on living,
though he possessed every other good thing."
—Aristotle

WHAT ARE THE ODDS?

It's been eleven weeks since my accident and I haven't had a pain-free day since then. I've had three weeks of physical therapy but I'm still stiff and sore most of the day and having difficulty sleeping through the night. I've got some pain in my right biceps that isn't noticeable except when I make certain motions. My solution has been to avoid those motions but I know I'll have to get it checked.

I can get stuff done in the mornings but my energy runs out by the afternoon. By evening all I can manage is to watch TV. Talk about useless! I need to work on gaining weight, which is hard because I don't have much of an appetite. I should gain back the ten pounds I've lost since the accident, not to mention the weight loss from the stem cell transplant.

In terms of my long-term health, I have a fifty/fifty chance of needing another bone marrow transplant within two years. I had an autologous transplant using my own cells, which removes the deadly possibility of graft-versus-host disease but has a higher likelihood of not working.

If I have to endure another transplant, I'll need a donor. If I can't find a match within my family I would join the seven thousand five hundred Americans who are actively searching the national registry for a donor at any given time. I would have about a sixty percent chance of finding a match since I'm Caucasian. If I were Hispanic the odds would drop to about forty-five percent, Asian to forty percent and African American to twenty-five percent. If I were of mixed race they would plummet even lower.

Donating Stem Cells
So I find myself becoming an advocate for bone marrow donations. It's a lifesaving gift. Most donations involve a simple peripheral blood stem cell draw, which is an outpatient, non-surgical procedure. Donors must be between eighteen and sixty years old and in good health. They can't be pregnant or have a medical condition such as cancer, severe arthritis or asthma, heart or autoimmune disease, or an STD. If you recently got a tattoo, you may have to wait a year to donate. You can get more info on the nuts and bolts of donating from the Be The Match FAQ web page.

If you're interested you can contact the Be The Match Registry Center near you. They'll have you complete a short health questionnaire and sign a consent form. Then they'll take a swab of cheek cells or a blood sample and your information will be added to a confidential donor database. The registration process can also be done online with a mail-in collection kit so you don't even have to leave home.

Donors and patients are matched according to tissue type, specifically their human leukocyte antigens (HLA). HLAs are proteins the immune system uses to recognize which cells are yours and which are foreign. The closer the HLA match, the better the chances of a successful transplant.

The best matches come from siblings or other family members who share DNA; people who don't have a suitable relative must find a donor in one of the bone marrow registries. While there are several million names in various databases around the world, it can be extremely difficult to find a viable match for a specific person, particularly for ethnic minorities and people of mixed ancestry.

If your HLA type matches someone needing a transplant, you'll be contacted about further testing. If the match is confirmed, you'll be asked to donate either peripheral blood stem cells or bone marrow depending on what's best for the patient. This is a volunteer process and you can withdraw at any time.

What a wise person once said about donating organs also applies to stem cells: "Don't think of organ donations as giving up part of yourself to keep a total stranger alive. It's really a total stranger giving up almost all of themselves to keep part of you alive."

Lawsuit to Save Lives

When I was diagnosed with cancer, filing a lawsuit that could help extend my life was the last thing on my mind. But in late October Susan and I travel to Washington, DC, to join a group of patients and a nonprofit called MoreMarrowDonors.Org. We're filing a constitutional challenge to a federal law that makes it a felony to offer compensation to marrow donors. We want to make it possible for MoreMarrowDonors.Org—of which I am a founding board member—to see if strategic incentives to the most needed donors will save lives.

The only means of changing the law available to the average citizen is the courts, so we are suing the Attorney General to be heard. The law at issue is the National Organ Transplant Act of 1984 (NOTA). NOTA was passed to prevent people from selling organs, like kidneys, which don't grow back. But stem cells from the bone marrow are a blood product. They regenerate within a matter of weeks so the donor loses nothing.

Donating stem cells is safe. I know; I've done it. It can be as simple as giving regular blood, although sometimes an unpleasant procedure is needed when marrow has to be extracted. In both cases incentives would probably make a real difference.

What we seek to do with the lawsuit is to strike down the federal restrictions on offering incentives as a way to expand the pool of bone marrow donors, thereby increasing the likelihood that more cancer sufferers will survive. The suit is the brainchild of the Institute for Justice in Arlington, Virginia. They're the ones spearheading the effort and bankrolling what will be a long fight in the courts. Jeff Rowes, lead attorney for IJ contacted me last spring about joining the suit and I readily agreed.

This is a multi-year process and whoever loses in the lower courts will push things all the way to the Supreme Court, if the justices will listen. I hope I'm around long enough to see the law changed.

o   o   o

"Laws are spider webs through which the big flies pass
and the little ones get caught."
—Honore de Balzac

PAIN AND PURPOSE

One hundred days since my accident and I'm back in Dr. Do's office on December 3 for more X-rays. Because of the ongoing pain and stiffness she sets me up with a physical trainer to get some new exercises. If these don't help I'll have to go back for more physical therapy. Either way I'm to come back in three months for evaluation.

As I go through December my shoulder gets worse, not better. Perhaps it's the exercises or the result of me doing more things like shoveling the drive or playing with the grandkids. My lower back is also sore, no doubt due to the increased activity. At least the cold doesn't seem to bother it. Thankfully I'm able to jog though. I'm up to thirty minutes a day.

A Greater Story
Donald Miller's book, *A Million Miles in a Thousand Years*, expands on the idea of life as story and explores how to live and tell a good one. Necessarily, some chapters deal with suffering. He paraphrases Holocaust survivor Victor Frankl, who believed that

> Suffering, as absurd as it seemed, pointed to a greater story in which, if one would only construe himself as a character within, he could find fulfillment in his tragic role, knowing

the plot was heading toward redemption. Such an understanding would take immense humility and immeasurable faith, a perspective perhaps achieved only in the context of near hopelessness.

In Frankl's thinking, pain indicated that life had meaning. "If one could have faith in something greater than himself, pain might be a path to experiencing a meaning beyond the false gratification of personal comfort."

In my thinking, pain is just pain sometimes. We hurt because we don't have a choice. The doctors don't know what's wrong. The medicines don't work. The circumstances can't be changed. Our bodies won't stop aging. The list goes on. Some pain is self-inflicted and we can learn to avoid it, but suffering isn't always an earned consequence; it's simply part of being human. It's universal, it's unrelenting and it stinks!

To keep from becoming a fatalist or nihilist, one has to assume—along with Frankl and Miller—that life is "heading toward redemption." When we can't find meaning in the suffering, we try to look beyond it to a higher purpose. But as noted, this takes "immense humility and immeasurable faith." And who has the energy for that when one is in pain? Souls more noble than me. All I can manage is to take one day at a time, to stay engaged with others and to hope that this life will all make sense in the next.

All attempts to ignore pain and suffering are fruitless; just ask the father of the Buddha. Still, most of us do all we can to avoid it. Except for those rare souls who embrace it and so take away some of its terror. Soul-numbing doubt didn't keep Mother Teresa from confronting human suffering at its worst. A generation before her, another humanitarian did the same, despite his pessimism. Albert Schweitzer won the 1952 Nobel Peace Prize for his humanitarian words and medical work in Africa. In his autobiography, *Out of My Life and Thought*, he writes,

> I am pessimistic because I feel the full weight of what we conceive to be the absence of purpose in the course of world events. Only at rare moments have I felt really glad to be alive. I cannot help but feel the suffering of all around me, not only of humanity but of the whole of creation.
>
> I have never tried to withdraw myself from this community of suffering. It seemed to me a matter of course that we should all take our share of the burden of pain that lies upon the world. Even while I was a boy at school it was clear to me that no explanation of the evil in the world could ever satisfy me; all explanations, I felt, ended in sophistries and at bottom had no other object than to minimize our sensitivity to the misery around us. ...
>
> But however concerned I was with the suffering in the world, I never let myself become lost in brooding over it. I always held firmly to the thought that each one of us can do a little to bring some portion of it to an end.

That last sentence is challenging enough to build an entire life on.

Therapists and Lawyers
As far as doing "a little to bring some portion of it [my own suffering] to an end," I've been in physical therapy for months now, with three different therapists and various approaches including manipulation, deep tissue massage and dry needling. I'm sure it's done some good but the underlying conditions still remain, as do the stiffness and pain. The disc at L-5 is still sixty percent compressed and my right

shoulder still has limited motion.

I see Dr. Do on February 23 for my six-month checkup and a final set of X-rays. Since there's nothing more to be done for me as an active patient she closes my account. Next month I'll go to Dr. Leppard, who will probably do the same. Then all my medical information will be forwarded to my attorney who will help me get enough insurance money to pay for everything. That process will probably take a few years, given our current legal system.

Although there's no question the other driver was at fault and her insurance is liable, that doesn't mean they will be in any hurry to settle. My attorney has warned me that we will probably have to file suit to get the full amount of her coverage. Insurance is a two-sided game. When you are the client paying the premiums, companies go out of their way to meet your every need. But if you become a claimant and are on the other side of a claim, everything slows down and the relationship becomes adversarial. Anything they have to pay out reduces their bottom line, which they are reluctant to do. Litigation often becomes necessary, not to get an inordinate sum but to collect up to the face value of the policy to cover expenses, which in my case will run into six figures when all the medical and legal fees are tallied.

In the meantime—or should I say "lean" time—I have to pay all expenses out of my own pocket.

o   o   o

"I know God will not give me anything I can't handle.
I just wish that He didn't trust me so much."
—Mother Teresa

OFF THE CUFF

R otator cuff that is. My right one has been bothering me since my accident last August. After months of unsuccessful physical therapy I finally had an MRI, which showed a "full tear in the supraspinatus tendon," the topmost of the four tendons that hold the shoulder in place and comprise the rotator cuff. According to ehealthMD.com,

> If a rotator cuff tendon becomes inflamed or is partially torn, it can cause pain and limit shoulder movement. If a tendon tears completely, the corresponding muscle can no longer affect movement of the arm. This type of injury usually causes severe limitations in shoulder movement as a result of pain and weakness.

I see Dr. Weinstein, a top orthopedic surgeon, and get scheduled for repair surgery on May 18. My right arm will be in a sling for several weeks and it will be many months before I regain full motion. Until then I will be "sinister."

Sinister is Latin for "left," as in left-handed. Someone who is right-handed would be referred to as "dexterous" or "deft." Obviously being different acquired the stigma of being evil or threatening. It's not much better in French, where a leftie would be called *gauche*, which also means awkward or lacking in social graces. The same negative bias exists in several other languages.

After surgery on my right shoulder, I will be going *gauche* for the next several weeks; joining the ten percent or so of the population that was born that way. And despite the connotations, I'll be in good company; four of our last five presidents have been left-handed. Two are Republicans and two are Democrats, so "handedness" isn't an indicator of political leaning:

» Ronald Reagan
» George H. W. Bush
» Bill Clinton
» Barack Obama

Other "sinister" world leaders:
» Alexander the Great
» Julius Caesar
» Charlemagne
» Napoleon Bonaparte
» Queen Victoria
» Benjamin Franklin

And when it comes to money, in 2006 researchers at Lafayette College and Johns Hopkins University found that right-handed men were fifteen percent poorer than left-handed men among those who attended college and twenty-six percent poorer if they graduated. The wage difference remains unexplained and also appears to apply to women.

I can only hope my income goes up during my next few months as a southpaw. (A "southpaw" is a left-handed pitcher whose pitching motion comes out of the south on most baseball diamonds, which have the batter facing east to avoid the afternoon sun.)

Post Op

Tuesday's surgery goes well as far as Dr. Weinstein is concerned. He repairs my rotator cuff and also fixes a tear in my biceps. The procedure is arthroscopic so I'll have no scars to show off, just two pin holes. The bruising is colorful but not very pervasive—another sign of a good surgeon.

The doc's been right about the post op pain; it's intense between pain pills. I trust he will also prove accurate about the healing process. I'll be in a sling for six weeks with an additional wraparound strap to further limit motion, including at night. I'll start physical therapy next Thursday, and if all goes well I should recover full range of motion in six to eight months.

If you want to experience life with a sling-and-strap and can't afford the hospital models—more expensive than a tuxedo—just make your own MacGyver Utility Sling. Empty your or your wife's favorite large purse and slice open the ends. Hang the straps over your neck and insert your arm up to the elbow. Now duct tape the sling to your body. Remove it to shower but be sure it's back on for bed. Sleeping in a sling eliminates all that random tossing and turning and gives you time to think about things other than sleep.

Fast forward a few weeks. Sleeping—or trying to—in a recliner is an exercise in futility. My heart goes out to people who have to do it every night like my sister-in-law, Linda. It's like being a conductor on a night train, with stops at 11:44, 12:47, 1:55, 3:07, 4:15 and 7:00.

Why a recliner? It hurts too much to lie flat for long, so a little angle helps offset the pull of gravity. Still, the pain gets me up every hour or so to stretch and start over. After the fact, I learned that rotator cuff repair is the most common surgery in America and one of the most painful. Not that I had much choice; surgery is the only viable way to fix a torn tendon.

One reason I'm telling you about my pain is that it's human

nature to crave both pity (for suffering) and praise (for bearing it so well). They are opposite ends of the same continuum—the need to be noticed. A few days ago at the coffee shop a lady commented on my sling. Not that she was impressed; she's had seventeen surgeries and counting. I also recently compared my post-op pics with those of Lance Armstrong's collarbone repair included in his book, *Comeback 2.0*. No contest.

I'm not bouncing back from surgery as fast as I'd hoped. The body doesn't like strangers rooting around with sharp instruments or injecting it with large doses of anesthesia. On the plus side, my bruising is coming along nicely. The hardest part is the constant fatigue. There seems to be more to it than the lack of sleep. At times I feel more drained than I did during chemo. The doctors have checked me over and run some tests but can't find an underlying cause.

Speaking of checkups, I get my one-year post transplant PET scan tomorrow (June 16) and will learn the results a week later. If the cancer is coming back anytime soon there should be some indication.

o   o   o

"I learned a long time ago that minor surgery
is when they do the operation on someone else, not you."
—Bill Walton

SIZE DOESN'T MATTER MUCH

I had my latest PET scan on Friday, June 18, and met with both my oncologist and my transplant surgeon the following Tuesday to go over the results. A few areas of concern on my previous scan cleared up but a few abdominal lymph nodes are showing low-grade activity. There's nothing large enough to biopsy or to give a clear diagnosis, but to be proactive I'm going to start a four-week course of chemo next Thursday.

This will be with the latest wonder drug—Rituxan, which I've had before. It has minimal side effects other than making me a little more vulnerable to infection. Rituxan is a monoclonal antibody, which according to the Mayo Clinic is "a laboratory-produced molecule that's carefully engineered to attach to specific defects in your cancer cells." Rituxan focuses on a protein called CD20 located on the surface of B-cells. It stimulates the immune system to eliminate these cancerous cells. In six months I'll repeat the Rituxan regime and get another scan. Hopefully it will be clean for the start of 2011.

The great value of a PET scan is the ability to detect suspicious activity on the cellular level. When it comes to tumors (that is, cancer), size doesn't matter that much. It's more about genetics. In a *New Yorker* article called "The Picture Problem," Malcolm

Gladwell interviewed several experts about the pros and cons of our current approach to early detection:

> The danger posed by a tumor is expressed visually. Large is bad; small is better—less likely to have metastasized. But here, too, tumors defy visual intuitions. According to Donald Berry of the M. D. Anderson Cancer Center in Houston, "We don't know whether it's tumor size that drives the metastatic process or whether all you need is a few million cells to start sloughing off to other parts of the body. We do observe that it's worse to have a bigger tumor. But not amazingly worse. The relationship is not as great as you'd think. ... Scientists discovered that even with tumors in the one-centimeter range ... the fate of the cancer seems already to have been set.

At its root, cancer is in the genes. We all produce defective ones but it's only when they get out of control that tumors sprout and cancer spreads. The best hope until we can find a genetic cure is to make our bodies a hostile environment for cancer through diet and lifestyle.

Genes may be the starting point for cancer but they don't have the last word. Dr. Servan-Schreiber says, "All research on cancer concurs. Genetic factors contribute to at most fifteen percent of mortalities from cancer. In short, there is no genetic fatality. We can all learn to protect ourselves."

Take breast cancer for example. Only between five and ten percent of the women who get breast cancer have the abnormal BRCA1 or BRCA2 genes. And more than ninety percent of those who have these genes don't get breast cancer.

People who do get cancer should not be fatalistic but realistic. The doctor goes on to stress

It must be stated at the outset that to date there is no alternative approach to cancer that can cure the illness. It is completely unreasonable to try to cure cancer without the best of conventional Western medicine: surgery, chemotherapy, radiation, immunotherapy, and soon, molecular genetics. At the same time, it is completely unreasonable to rely only on this purely technical approach and neglect the natural capacity of our bodies to protect against tumors. We can take advantage of this natural protection to either prevent the disease or enhance the benefits of treatment.

As I head into my third year with cancer, my survival strategy is fourfold:
  » advanced medical treatment
  » aggressive natural protection
  » all the prayer I can get
  » attending church regularly

Survival of the Religious

According to research cited by Ben Sherwood in his book *The Survivors Club: Secrets and Science That Could Save Your Life*, "people who go to church regularly live around *seven years longer* than people who don't. ... More precisely, if you go to church once a week, your advantage is 6.6 years. If you worship at church more than once a week, your edge increases to 7.6 years, a bonus of one additional year."

It's not clear whether the particular religion matters, says Dr. Harold Koenig of Duke University Medical Center. More research is needed to determine if the effects are the same for Christianity, Buddhism, Islam, Judaism or any other creed. However, longer life appears to be correlated with the extent to which faith is integrated into daily decisions and actions. People with committed religious beliefs tend to have stronger support systems and more solid relationships; they are more likely to follow teachings that reinforce a healthier lifestyle.

If religion prolongs your life; what about the opposite? What if you're struggling with your faith like me? Once more the answer is stunning. It turns out that wrestling with God could kill you! An extensive study by Dr. Kenneth Pargament showed that grappling with God put patients at increased risk of death.

> More precisely, patients in religious turmoil had a six to ten percent greater risk of dying compared to those who weren't. … Patients who felt alienated from or unloved by God and attributed their illness to the devil were nineteen to twenty-eight percent more likely to die during the two-year study period.

Perhaps my belief in an Almighty God and my questions about what he's up to in my life cancel each other out where longevity is concerned.

At least I'm still getting the Church Attendance bump.

o   o   o

"All right, I'm still alive;
what do I do now?"
—Stephen Wright

INVOLUNTARY RECIDIVISM

Recidivism means "a tendency to relapse into a previous condition or mode of behavior; especially relapse into criminal behavior." In my case it's medical behavior. That's why I'm back in the Memorial Cancer Center for four weekly Rituxan treatments. Rituxan has dramatically improved the long-term outcomes for B-cell lymphoma patients. It's so effective that some oncologists feel it's tantamount to malpractice not to prescribe it.

On our second weekly visit to the outpatient clinic someone asks Susan if I'm her father. The solace I take from looking older is that people may suspect I'm rich and she's a trophy wife. I'm not rich but Susan is a prize beyond compare!

I lose a few more pounds this month as my nausea and fatigue continue. I'm trying to get an appointment with a recommended GI doctor to see if he can find a cause for my maladies but his earliest opening is in August. I'm getting more sleep but becoming more tired. This is "can't get out of the chair" fatigue, and if it doesn't improve Dr. Dax will send me for some tests.

Ill Humored

The Greeks and Romans had a "humorist" view of the body that held sway from Hippocrates into the nineteenth century. Essentially, this approach taught that the human body was filled with four basic substances called "humors."

Humor	Season	Element	Organ	Qualities	Name	Characteristics
blood	spring	air	liver	warm and moist	sanguine	courageous, hopeful, amorous
yellow bile	summer	fire	gall bladder	warm and dry	choleric	easily angered, bad tempered
black bile	autumn	earth	spleen	cold and dry	melancholic	despondent, sleepless, irritable
phlegm	winter	water	brain/ lungs	cold and moist	phlegmatic	calm, unemotional

All diseases and disabilities resulted from an excess or deficit of one of these four. When a patient was suffering from a surplus or imbalance of one fluid, then his or her personality and physical health would be affected. We still use these terms to describe basic temperaments: sanguine, choleric, melancholic and phlegmatic.

I've been in ill-humor for the past few months and can't figure out the cause. It's something more than the surgery, which was hard enough. I've had several scans and tests and everything is normal, yet something is out of balance. If it keeps up I'm going to slide down the table from sanguine to melancholic. And with enough Percocet, I could make it all the way to phlegmatic!

In my quest to find a cause, I had myself tested for celiac disease. A friend who knew of my symptoms suggested the diagnosis and the nurse practitioner at the clinic confirmed it as a possible culprit in my case.

When people with celiac disease eat foods containing gluten, it results in damage to the finger-like villi of the small intestines. Left untreated, it can cause further complications such as autoimmune diseases, osteoporosis, thyroid disease and cancer.

Celiac disease can be difficult to diagnose because it manifests itself in a variety of ways. The only treatment is a lifelong gluten-free diet. One interesting aspect is that celiac can be dormant until triggered by physical trauma. In my case I have several to choose from, surgery being the most recent.

False alarm.

My tests come back negative, for which I'm very thankful. Gluten is not my enemy, which means I still need to find the root of my malaise. The next step is seeing a GI doc. If he can't find anything, the fatigue and queasiness may just be the cumulative result of the last two years of trauma. In that case the only cure is time.

And healthy eating, which includes bucking the grisly habit adversely affecting most Americans—including me: eating too much red meat. *Mother Jones* reports,

> Americans eat about eight ounces of meat every day, more than twice the rest of the world's average. … In 2009, a landmark National Cancer Institute study of 500,000 Americans between the ages of 50 and 71 found that people who eat a quarter-pound of red meat or processed meat every day were 30 percent more likely to die in the 10 years of the study than those who ate 5 ounces of red meat or less per week.

If we broaden the scope to include non-red meat, one study cited in *Time* (08/23/10) concludes that the average American will consume a total of twenty-one thousand animals. So much meat consumption is bad for our bodies and worse for our planet. According to a 2006 United Nations' report, one-third of Earth's arable land is devoted to growing animal feed. Animal farming is responsible for sixty-five percent of nitrous oxide emissions, a gas that contributes to global warming almost three hundred times more than carbon dioxide. And the methane omitted by cows due to their high-corn diet contributes to global warming twenty-three times more than CO^2.

That's right; cow farts may be doing more damage than car exhaust.

If you're concerned about the environment and can't afford a hybrid car, skip a few Big Macs. If you're concerned about your own internal combustion engine, cut down on the *carne*.

o   o   o

"Life expectancy would grow by leaps and bounds
if green vegetables smelled as good as bacon."
—Doug Larson

CANDID CAMERA

Because of my stomach problems, I go in for an EGD procedure on August 16. EGD stands for esophagogastroduodenoscopy, aka upper endoscopy. It is just as invasive as a colonoscopy but not as embarrassing. I have no idea how much it will cost; I only hope it helps find the problem.

The doctor sprays a numbing medication into the back of my throat, inserts an endoscope (a bendable tube that acts as a camera) and examines my esophagus, stomach and small intestine for any growths or foreign bodies. Fortunately they give me Versed, which creates amnesia, and Fentanyl, which is an analgesic. Together they cause conscious sedation or "twilight sleep," so although I am awake during the procedure, I don't remember it.

The results come back on Friday, August 20. I have some erythema, or irritation, of the esophagus and stomach. No suggestion in the report as to what's causing it and the only treatment recommended is to take antacid tablets and to stop eating most foods. The good news is there's nothing else wrong. The bad news is I still feel queasy and have no idea why. My diet didn't change, so what's causing the problem? It started after my shoulder surgery; go figure. Susan thinks it's a byproduct of all I've been through the past year.

Probiotics

Since my shoulder surgery in May, I've been to my oncologist, a GP, an NP and a GI specialist seeking to find the cause of my fatigue and digestive troubles—without results. So I've added Dr. Christie, a chiropractor/nutritionist, to the list. She's helping me take a more holistic look at my lifestyle and diet with the goal of getting my major systems into better shape. Among other things, she gets me started on probiotics to counter the various antibiotics I've been taking for more than two years. Web MD gives the following definition:

> Probiotics are bacteria that help maintain the natural balance of organisms (microflora) in the intestines camera. The normal human digestive tract contains about 400 types of probiotic bacteria that reduce the growth of harmful bacteria and promote a healthy digestive system. The largest group of probiotic bacteria in the intestine is lactic acid bacteria, of which Lactobacillus acidophilus, found in yogurt with live cultures, is the best known. Yeast is also a probiotic substance. Probiotics are also available as dietary supplements (http://www.webmd.com/digestive-disorders/tc/probiotics-topic-overview).

The Mayo Clinic says, "You don't necessarily need probiotics to be healthy. However, these microorganisms may help with digestion and offer protection from harmful bacteria, just as the existing 'good' bacteria in your body already do." I'm taking two kinds of probiotics. Not sure if they're helping but they can't hurt.

While I'm on the subject of diet, let me say that outside of school, Ds are good for you and you might want to add some to your health report card. Dr. David Servan-Schreiber notes,

> Substantial scientific evidence now exists supporting the role of vitamin D in prevention of cancer. Multiple research findings

have reasonably established that an adequate serum vitamin D status is independently associated with substantially lower incidence rates of several types of cancer, including breast, colon, ovary, non-Hodgkin lymphoma [the kind I have] and several other types.

The appropriate intake of vitamin D for cancer risk reduction depends on the individual's age, skin type, lifestyle, and latitude of residence. Recent scientific evidence indicates that intakes of 1000–2000 IU per day could prevent a substantial proportion of cancers and would also be effective in reducing risks of falls, fractures, heart diseases and strokes, multiple sclerosis and type I childhood diabetes.

My family physician put me on vitamin D months ago for my general health; I'm encouraged to learn of its cancer-fighting properties.

Bottom Line: aDD more "D" to your Diet.

Don't Delay!

Anticancer Rules
Dr. Servan-Schreiber recently had a piece in the Huffington Post called *20 New Anticancer Rules*. Here are the ones I've found especially helpful:

Food Rules:
1. Go retro: Your main course should be 80 percent vegetables, 20 percent animal protein, like it was in the old days.
4. Spice it up: Add turmeric (with black pepper) when cooking. This yellow spice is the most powerful natural anti-inflammatory agent.
5. Skip the potato: Potatoes raise blood sugar, which can feed inflammation and cancer growth.

7. Remember not all eggs are created equal: Choose only omega-3 eggs, or don't eat the yolks.

12. Make room for exceptions. What matters is what you do on a daily basis, not the occasional treat.

Non-Food Rules:

1. Get physical: Make time to exercise, be it walking, dancing or running. Aim for 30 minutes of physical activity at least 5 days a week.

4. Reach out to at least two friends for support (logistical and emotional) during times of stress, even if it's through the Internet. But if they're within arm's reach, go ahead and hug them, often!

7. Cultivate happiness like a garden: Make sure you do one thing you love for yourself on most days (it doesn't have to take long).

o   o   o

A Short History of Medicine:

2000 B.C. "Here, eat this root."

1000 B.C. "That root is heathen, say this prayer."

1850 A.D. "That prayer is superstition, drink this potion."

1940 A.D. "That potion is snake oil, swallow this pill."

1985 A.D. "That pill is ineffective, take this antibiotic."

2000 A.D. "That antibiotic is artificial. Here, eat this root."

—Author Unknown

TEMPORARY CONDITION

Monday, September 13, is my follow-up with the doctor who did my shoulder surgery. I've only recovered about sixty percent of my range of motion due to the formation of scar tissue. Dr. Weinstein says this level of adhesion occurs only in one percent of his patients. Just my luck.

I'll do six more weeks of aggressive physical therapy. If things don't improve, he can go back in and remove the scar tissue. Afterwards I wouldn't be immobilized in a sling but would start PT right away. This will be even more painful than what I've already been through but should produce better results. The other option would be to settle for a limited range of motion the rest of my life—an alternative that seems pretty good some days compared to the pain of therapy and another surgery.

For more than two years now I've lived with pain of varying severity, from annoying to almost dead. Through it all, I still choose to believe life is a gift to be opened and enjoyed each new day—suffering and all.

Light The Night
My shoulder and back give me problems but my legs work fine, so this year I'm able to participate in Light The Night in downtown

Colorado Springs on Thursday, September 23. This is the annual fundraising event for the Leukemia & Lymphoma Society (LLS). September is Blood Cancer Awareness Month and LLS celebrates with Light The Night walks that honor lives touched by cancer and raise support for the search to find cures.

For more than sixty years, LLS has been focused on people with blood cancers. It is the largest foundation of its kind in the country and has no shortage of work to do as someone is diagnosed with a blood cancer every four minutes. Last year, LLS researchers conducted more than ninety clinical trials, a critical step in the development of new treatments and cures that will help patients like me live better, longer lives.

In addition to funding vital research, the society also provides grants to assist patients with medical costs. As the recipient of a few of these grants, I know how helpful they can be. This year alone they will

» invest $72 million, which includes funding for 103 new grants to researchers and $8 million in contracts through the LLS Therapy Acceleration Program;
» support 347 research projects in the United States and ten other countries;
» provide financial assistance to patients like me;
» sponsor scientific conferences around the country;
» produce educational materials and videos;
» run dozens of Family Support Groups nationwide.

Cancer survivors get white T-shirts; the rest of the supporters wear red ones. Lots of folks are walking on behalf of friends and loved ones who lost their battle with cancer. One lady in front of me has two "In Memory" patches on her shoulders; one for her husband and another for her daughter. She herself is wearing a survivor T-shirt—and most amazingly, a smile.

Death and Life

On Tuesday, September 28, I get the results of my most recent PET scan. No sign of cancer ... for now, which officially puts me in remission. I know it can be a temporary condition, but then life itself is a temporary condition. I'm thankful for every day I get.

I ascribe my improvement to a healthier diet and the Rituxan chemo (next round coming up in January). I suspect prayer plays a part and I appreciate all I can get. I still can't pray for myself very well; my head gets in the way of my heart.

In *The Devil's Dictionary*, Ambrose Bierce has the following definition: "Pray—to ask that the laws of the universe be annulled in behalf of a single petitioner confessedly unworthy." This strikes me as accurate, as far as it goes. Cause and effect are hard-wired into creation (except on the quantum level) and can't be short-circuited. What makes prayer work—when it does—is the act of God being God. Who is to tell him what he can and can't do? Still, I doubt he tinkers with our circumstances nearly as often as we think, which makes me reluctant to ask.

Living with a potentially terminal disease has caused me to make eye contact with death. It's not a pleasant experience and one that most of us avoid as long as possible. Few in our death-defying culture want to face our mortality.

An attorney friend of mine has written some great materials to help older people plan for death and younger people prepare for new fiduciary responsibilities. One tool he's compiled to drive home the reality that life comes with an expiration date is a Death Calendar. It has the sobering caption, "These Notable People Never Thought They Would Die Either ...."

It's sobering to flip through the months and find the rich, the powerful, the famous—the deceased. No date is blank, "for death is the destiny of every man; the living should take this to heart" (Ecclesiastes 7:2). Do you believe this means your death date is as

MIKE HAMEL

certain as your birth date? Does the future already exist? And if so, can our choices and actions change it in any way?

When Nobel laureate Isaac Bashevis Singer was asked if he believed in free will, he responded, "I have no choice."

The ranks of those who insist on a fixed future include many Christians (especially Calvinists), Muslims and Jews. Many secular determinists and noted scientists (including Einstein) believe the future is as unchangeable as the past. This immutability is deduced from the character of God in the case of the former and the laws of classical physics in the case of the latter.

And yet, while millions believe in a fixed future, no one *behaves* as if it's the way things are. We all live as though we have real choices that matter. Do you pray? If the future is set, whether you pray or not can't change it: unless of course you were predestined to pray, in which case you had no free will in choosing to do so. Do you work out, watch your diet, wear a seatbelt? Why bother if the dates that will appear on your tombstone have already been chiseled in (Psalm 139:16)?

We bother to pray and to take care of ourselves because we instinctively believe choices have consequences. We think what we do today will affect tomorrow. Delusion or reality, we cannot live otherwise.

o   o   o

"Life is a terminal disease,
and it is sexually transmitted."
—John Cleese

146

SYSTEM REBOOT

One byproduct of my bone marrow transplant last year was the destruction of my immune system. It was wiped clean by the high-dose chemo and rebooted by the infusion of my own stem cells. But like a computer that's been turned off and on, it didn't retain any RAM (Random Access Memory). All my childhood vaccinations and a lifetime of acquired immunities were erased. I have to begin again at the beginning, which is what takes me to the outpatient clinic at Memorial Hospital on Tuesday, October 14, for the first in a series of re-inoculations. I get a salvo of six shots—three in each arm—to protect me from polio, measles, mumps, rubella, diphtheria, tetanus, hepatitis B, pneumonia and influenza.

I don't feel so hot for a few days afterward; I wonder why? I wish there was a vaccine for the common cold. I've had several this year another side effect of a pristine immune system.

Back to Square One
Aggressive physical therapy didn't improve my shoulder so I head back to the operating room on Tuesday, November 23, for the sixth time in the last two years—four port surgeries and two shoulder operations. Dr. Weinstein will use an arthroscopic scalpel to scrape out excessive scar tissue that's formed since my first shoulder surgery

last May. Physical therapy will start the next day to keep the scar tissue from reforming.

I *am not* looking forward to going through it all again at a more intense level: sharp pain, nights in the recliner, aggressive physical therapy. Hopefully I won't have the same stomach issues. But I *am* looking forward to regaining full motion with my right arm; the better to play with my grandkids and to resume dance lessons with Susan next year. Look for our new reality show, *Dancing with the Scars!*

The surgery takes longer than expected, as does regaining my senses in the recovery room. The doctor eventually comes by and tells me there was a lot of adhesion to remove. He also says my original tear had not completely healed (or else was re-torn) and he had to repair it again.

I'm sent home sporting a new piece of equipment—a nerve block catheter. When I sit, my right hand lays sound asleep in my lap. When I stand, it hangs by my side like a three-foot kielbasa. I wonder if this is anything like what a paraplegic feels—or doesn't feel to be precise. In my case I would be a monoplegic.

The device docs what it says, interrupts the nerve impulses between arm and brain. The blocking agent is a drug called ropivacaine, aka Naropin. Ropivacaine is a local anesthetic causing loss of feeling during surgical procedures, labor and delivery, or for short-term pain management. It definitely blocks out the pain, along with all other sensation, which is comforting. What is ominous is why they chose to use it this time. Dr. Weinstein did a lot of cutting and scraping and I suppose my shoulder will be doing a lot of moaning and groaning about it.

At my post-op visit on Friday I'm ordered back into a sling for six weeks. No active arm movement allowed, just what they call aggressive passive physical therapy. Having to start over really refries my beans. Why didn't the tear heal? Have cancer and chemo messed up my recuperative powers? Or did I re-tear the tendon trying to stretch out the scar tissue as instructed? Whatever the cause, I'm back to square one with my shoulder. And if I don't move my arm, what's to keep me from getting the same poor results as the first time around?

After the doctor's office I have to speak at the funeral of my mom's second husband. Since Del was a retired air force veteran he's buried with full military honors at Fort Logan National Cemetery in Denver. My mom's urn, which has been at my sister's house for six years, is there to be interred with his. I can barely get through my part of the service as the memories and the ritual bring me to tears. Latter I put the scene into these words:

> Awash in an ocean of simple white tombstones,
>   sit two wooden boxes at rest side by side;
> a folding of colors, a volley of rifles
>   and squadrons of geese in commemorative flight.

o   o   o

"We cannot forecast anything about the future for certain;
any attempt of our fantasy to fill the emptiness
with wish-fulfilling concreteness
is more a sign of weak faith than of strong hope.
Faith asks us to jump; to surrender and believe that
somewhere, somehow, someone will catch us and bring us home."
—Henri Nouwen

ROAD TO RECOVERY

Baby boomers will remember the band Three Dog Night. Well, my post-op routine in December involves a Three Bed Night that goes something like this: I adjust my sling, pop four ibuprofen and a Lunesta, and assume the position in my regular bed. It's only a few minutes until my shoulder starts squawking. I'll listen for a while to be polite but when the pain gets too much I slip out of bed, saying good night to Susan, and slide into the small recliner for a nap. A decent one lasts two or three hours. The narrow seat doesn't allow for the tossing and turning that's good for sleep but bad for a shoulder repair.

Whenever I wake up I transfer to the big recliner, which is a bit roomier but still keeps me strictly supine. I have a traveling blanket and pillow I take with me, along with a warm pair of socks. Sometimes I walk around and stretch the kinks out of my arm. This nocturnal migration is driven by pain. It should last another six-or-eight weeks if I remember correctly. (What I didn't remember too well was how much it hurts!) This time around, though, instead of my three stops being in different parts of the house, I have all my resting places in one room.

I suffer ... I learn ... I adapt.

And I take pills. I've taken hundreds over the past thirty months: vitamins and supplements, antibiotics and probiotics, antiemetics and analgesics, steroids and sleep aids and, most reluctantly, narcotics and painkillers. For some reason these are the hardest for me to swallow. I don't know if it's the male psyche or a misguided machismo but I balk at taking pain pills.

Susan can't figure out why I would rather suffer than take the Percocet I've been given for my shoulder and I can't explain it to her because there's no good reason. Maybe it's a twisted form of resistance, of standing up to the attacker, of not wanting to admit I can't handle the pain. How stupid is that!

Percocet is a brand name for a combination of oxycodone (a narcotic) and acetaminophen (Tylenol). Oxycodone is an opiate similar to morphine, which means it can be habit-forming. Percocet is a schedule II narcotic that packs more punch than, say, Vicodin, a schedule III narcotic with hydrocodone, but it isn't as potent as schedule I drugs like heroin and cocaine. Addiction to oxycodone can be dangerous, as Anna Nicole Smith, Heath Ledger, Michael Jackson and other celebrities failed to appreciate. But one pill every few nights doesn't concern me.

The other pill I'm taking that can be habit forming is Lunesta. The active ingredient—eszopiclone—is in a class of drugs called hypnotics. No one knows exactly how eszopiclone works but it's thought to slow the brain down by interacting with GABA (gamma-aminobutyric acid) receptors. I just know it helps me sleep. I've been on and off it a few times during chemo and my transplant so I'm not worried about snubbing the little blue pills again when the time comes.

I wish I could take a pill that would restore a sense of general wellbeing. The combination of lack of sleep and constant pain makes me feel out of focus most days. This chronic state of dis-ability wears down the body and mind. It shortens my effective workday by about half and makes it difficult to keep active and stay positive.

The Weinstein Report

On December 27 I see Dr. Weinstein for the first time since my shoulder surgery five weeks ago. Progress is slow but he thinks I'll gain more mobility with several more months of physical therapy. I've used up all the PT my insurance will cover and he graciously says his staff will treat me for free until my new plan starts in February.

Dr. Weinstein tells me to wear the sling for one more week, at least when I'm up and about. He also reveals how to avoid wearing it to bed. Put on a T-shirt and keep your sore arm by your side instead of sticking it through the armhole. This keeps you from flailing. I've included this piece of expert medical advice in my book at no extra charge because that's the kind of caring author I am.

I've been going to PT—usually twice a week—and doing stretching exercises at home—usually twice a day—for more than a year now. It's gotten very old. Having someone crank your body where it doesn't want to go is an unpleasant experience. It's made tolerable by the winsome personality of the dungeon master, Dave. He *says* he doesn't like to hurt me but he usually has a smile on his face when I have tears in my eyes.

The scar tissue seems to be building up as fast as before and I'm not sure how much benefit I'll realize from the second surgery. (I am daily aware of the cost, though.) Whatever range of motion I end up with will have to suffice. I will not do another surgery. If I knew two months ago what I know now, I don't think I would have done the second one.

Best-case scenario: I'd like to be able to lift my right arm high enough to resume ballroom dancing lessons.

o   o   o

"Never argue with a doctor;
he has inside information."
—Bob Elliot

TALE OF TWO MIKES

Mike Rogers and I had a lot in common. Both of us had moved
away from fundamentalist roots in our quest for a deeper
understanding of God. Both of us were pastors. Both of us were
diagnosed with NHL the same month and endured similar chemo
regimes and relapses. Subsequently we both underwent stem cell
transplants about a month apart in the summer of 2009.

We kept in touch and on June 25, 2010, Mike commented on
my blog:

> Mike, I'm sympathetic. I'm in the hospital for 5 days right
> now getting some more chemo because my lymphoma has
> come back with a vengeance. I'm having R-EPOCH, and
> talking of having the radioimmunotherapy drug Bexxar fol-
> lowing. Have been and will continue to pray for you.

We were kindred spirits and took similar attitudes toward our
suffering. The day after the above post he wrote,

> It's been a long ride and I've stayed pretty even keeled spiritu-
> ally and emotionally. I realized a long time ago not much of
> this is in my hands, though a pleasant and hopeful attitude is

no doubt helpful. I pretty much just do what I need to day after day and wait on the Lord's will.

Praying for you.

Mike sent me an encouraging note on October 12, 2010. Then on January 10, 2011, I heard from his wife:

This is from Deb, Mike's wife. My Mike is now free from his lymphoma having passed from this life on 12/25/2010 at 12:25 a.m. We were able on the 15th of December to return to Colorado, and he delighted in the care and bosom of our family for the last 10 days.

What a courageous soul he was, and never a single "why me!" We miss him greatly, but are so happy he is at last free. Only one year ago he was recovering from his stem cell transplant. I know he'd want me to let you know. We followed your transplant story here, just ahead of his. Praise God for your clean scan.

With so much in common—positive attitudes, quality medical care, loving families, passionate prayers—why was the outcome different for us? The odds of long-term survival after a stem cell transplant are about fifty/fifty. But who or what determines on which side of the "/" we find ourselves?

The *mechanics* of life and death are a matter of genetics, lifestyle and chance. The *meaning* of it all is something only God knows, and he's not very forthcoming with details this side of the grave.

In the absence of answers we are left with faith and hope. "Now faith is confidence in what we hope for and assurance about what we do not see" (Hebrews 11:1). My confidence in faith has been shaken by what I've learned and experienced in the past few years. But I still cling to hope.

Survival

My latest PET scan came back clean, for which I am profoundly thankful. Still, I have four weeks of Rituxan chemo next month (January 2011), and more rounds of the stuff in July. It's part of a two-year regime to keep the lymphoma at bay. I'm uncomfortable with the word "remission," and I don't believe cancer can be "cured." Its lethal aggression can be slowed and even halted for long periods but eradicated from our genes—I doubt it. When people ask about my condition I tell them I still have cancer but it currently doesn't have me. I suspect it will get me in the end, but everyone has to die of something.

The chief milestone on most cancer journeys is overall survivability (OS), which is five years. I'm halfway there. Thanks to recent medical advances, almost seventy percent of NHL patients live past their OS date. There are no guarantees in life, though. You could get hit by a car on your way to the oncologist.

The aftereffects of my auto accident will last the rest of my days. My ribs and sternum have healed but my L5 disc will stay sixty percent compressed and deteriorate with time. I'm still in physical therapy for my shoulder and don't know what range of motion I'll regain in the end. (My pessimistic guess is about seventy-five percent.) I haven't had a pain-free day since August 25, 2009, and as far as nights go, I'm still taking Lunesta and catnapping in recliners. But I've had great medical care and I'm learning to adapt to my limitations.

I have experienced more physical pain in the last thirty months than in my previous fifty-five years combined. I've chosen to write about it in a casual, almost flippant, manner at times but this doesn't change the fact that *it hurts!* From the systemic torment of a stem cell transplant to the serrated torture of two shoulder surgeries I've been through several octaves on the pain scale. White keys and black. Major chords and minor.

Parts of my background score might sound familiar to many of you. You or a loved one may have cancer; you may face other physical challenges; or you may be hounded by spiritual doubts and questions. We are all players in the same orchestra. The best we can hope for is that

- » what sometimes seems like a blaring cacophony is really a grand symphony of beautiful complexity.
- » whether we're playing a kettle drum or a piccolo, our small parts fit somehow into the whole piece.
- » even when we can't see him, there's a Maestro on the podium who knows what he's doing.

I would not have chosen the composition I've been given to play—not that I was asked. Most times I feel woefully out of tune, but I choose to stay engaged and to keep learning. At the beginning of a new year I choose to raise my glass along with Tevye and his friends and drink To Life!

o   o   o

Life has a way of confusing us,
blessing and bruising us,
Drink l'chaim, to life!
God would like us to be joyful,
even when our hearts lie panting on the floor.
How much more can we be joyful,
when there's really something to be joyful for?
To life, to life, l'chaim!

To us and our good fortune!
Be happy, be healthy, long life!
And if our good fortune never comes,
Here's to whatever comes,
Drink l'chaim, to life!
—"Fiddler on the Roof"

PART IV
THE LONG SHADOW
JANUARY 2011 – DECEMBER 2012

"Once you've had cancer
you're always in the waiting room."
—George Carlin

RITUXAN REGIME

On January 7, 2011, I get the results of my latest PET scan—*clean*! No sign of cancer! It's my second clear scan in a row, which ties my personal best. Still, I find myself in the Memorial Health Spa, aka Outpatient Chemo Clinic, for the first of four weekly rounds of wonder drugs. Not your idea of a health spa?

» The treatment is ridiculously expensive.
» I am pampered by a highly trained staff.
» I have a certain "glow" after treatment.

Like every other day in the clinic, the morning starts with a blood test to make sure I'm healthy enough for the planned festivities. Next come Benadryl and Ativan in a preemptive strike against nausea. A saline drip is started to keep me hydrated.

The star of this show is Rituxan, one of the fabled "magic bullets" in the field of oncology. The Mayo Clinic describes this monoclonal antibody "as a laboratory-produced molecule that's carefully engineered to attach to specific defects in your cancer cells. Monoclonal antibodies mimic the antibodies your body naturally produces as part of your immune system's response to germs, vaccines and other invaders." I get seventy milligrams of it dripped in over several hours.

Targeting the attack on cancer in this way reduces many of the side effects of broad-based chemotherapy that damage healthy tissues. Chemo drugs don't restore, they destroy. And the most potent aren't administered in pill form or syringes. They come in bags!

Rituxan doesn't make me feel as bad as some of the other chemo treatments I've had. No projectile vomiting or mandatory hospitalization. Still, it's not a recreational drug I would recommend, especially at more than $10,000 a dose.

Heard the One about . . . ?

There is nothing funny about cancer but I find it helps to maintain a sense of humor. Humor Therapy is even encouraged by the American Cancer Society as

> A complementary method to promote health and cope with illness. ... Humor has physical effects because it can stimulate the circulatory system, immune system, and other systems in the body. ... The physical effects of laughter on the body include increased breathing, increased oxygen use, short-term changes in hormones and certain neurotransmitters, and increased heart rate. Many hospitals and treatment centers have set up special rooms with humorous materials for the purpose of making people laugh, such as movies, audio recordings, books, games, and puzzles.

There aren't too many funny cancer jokes but these aren't bad:

> A man isn't feeling well, so he goes to his doctor. The doctor examines him, then asks to speak with his wife. The doctor tells the wife her husband has cancer. The wife asks, "Can he be cured?"
> The doctor replies, "There's a chance we can cure him with

chemotherapy, but you will need to take care of him every day for the next year—cooking all the meals, cleaning up the vomit, changing the bed pan, driving him to the hospital for daily treatments, and so on."

When the wife comes out to the waiting room, the husband asks her what the doctor said. The wife answers, "He said that you're going to die."

Have you ever noticed nobody has ever ordered a grapefruit the size of a tumor? Ever. There's no reciprocity. —Janeane Garofalo

Cancer cures smoking—eventually.

Doctor: The tests show that your cancer is advanced. You have six months to live.
Patient: But, doc, I can't pay off my medical bills in six months.
Doctor: In that case, you have six months more. —Syd Love

You've been a great audience. I'll be playing the Memorial Outpatient Clinic again in July.

Wartime Survivors

I've had some pain and numbness on the left side of my neck and jaw for months now. I've seen a doctor, dentist, ENT specialist and physical therapist but no one can figure out what's wrong. So on May 3 I have a CT scan to check my lymph nodes. This involves drinking about a quart of contrast that tastes like puréed sheetrock. The scan is painless and only takes a few minutes as opposed to a few hours for a PET scan.

When I get the results on Thursday, the swelling turns out to be the parotid gland instead of a lymph node, which means my lymphoma hasn't returned. My oncologist has no idea what's causing the pain and numbness but he doesn't suspect cancer.

The CT scan revealed no suspicious cervical, pelvic, supraclavicular axillary, or medastinal lymphadenopathy. The full body scan also shows my major organs and arteries to be in good shape. One negative is that my spine shows some degeneration, probably due to my accident.

I'm still alive and kicking on June 5, which is National Cancer Survivor Day (NCSD). I'm one of twelve million American survivors of the Big C and not among its six hundred thousand US victims last year. The NCSD Foundations defines a survivor as "anyone living with a history of cancer—from the moment of diagnosis through the remainder of life." That definition applies to all sorts of other stressful situations: deadly disease, debilitating accident, dysfunctional family, broken marriage, death of a child, widowhood, financial ruin.

I spend the third weekend in June in Washington, DC, where I participate in a conference sponsored by the Institute for Justice (IJ), the organization behind the lawsuit seeking to change the law governing bone marrow donations.

My involvement with groups like the Institute for Justice, More Marrow Donors and the Leukemia & Lymphoma Society is how I participate as a foot soldier in the war on cancer. It was forty years ago in this very city that President Nixon signed the National Cancer Act and declared war on the disease. The law earmarked $1.5 million for research over three years and made the fight a national priority. The stated goal was to cure cancer by the Bicentennial (1976). The actual results have been discouraging, as oncologist Dr. David Agus notes in *The End of Illness*:

> Since signing of the National Cancer Act of 1971, we've lost more than 12 million Americans to cancer. Every time a

citizen pays $10 in taxes, only one penny goes to cancer re-search; we allocate less that $5 billion yearly for cancer research while Americans spend $20 billion a year on beauty products, and $5.3 billion on potato chips! We lose roughly 560,000 people a year to cancer, which is 160,000 more than lost their lives in World War II.

I have friends who are losing their battle with cancer. Statistics are boring and irrelevant—until the numbers represent those you love.

o   o   o

"Statistics are human beings with the tears wiped off."
—Paul Brodeur

NEW CANCER

It doesn't show on the outside but my emotions are more fragile since the call from the clinic last Thursday (August 17) saying the lump on my neck was cancerous. Not lymphoma this time and it will take a PET/CT to determine exactly what I'm up against. Probably one of those secondary cancers brought on by heavy chemo or a latent genetic variety come to the fore since my immune system's been suppressed for so long.

Fast-forward a few days and the PET scan results reveal a new cancer wrapped in a mystery. I have squamous cell carcinoma in the lymph node below my left ear. The tumor isn't caused by lymphoma, which is good. But squamous cell carcinoma is a skin cancer, which means it came from somewhere else. However, the scan didn't detect cancer anywhere else, hence the mystery. My own theory is that it's a brain tumor that got lost.

I will have more tests to search for the source and undergo surgery in a few weeks to remove the lymph node and parotid gland under my cheek. Follow-up will include radiation and chemo. I'm pretty discouraged. Three cancers in three years.

Omne Trium Perfectum is Latin for "everything that comes in threes is perfect," or, "every set of three is complete." In common parlance it's known as The Rule of Three.

The "rule of three" is a principle in writing that suggests that things that come in threes are inherently funnier, more satisfying, or more effective than other numbers of things. ... A series of three is often used to create a progression in which the tension is created, then built up, built up even more, and finally released (http://en.wikipedia.org/wiki/Rule_of_three_%28writing%29).

I'm facing my third cancer in three years. I have recently undergone three tests to confirm the cancer. I have three doctors who are collaborating on my case. There is nothing "perfect" about the Rule of Three when it comes to cancer. I can only hope my set of three is "complete."

Pneumonia and Parotidectomy
As if the cancer isn't enough, I contract pneumonia the third week of August. It has really wiped me out. I haven't felt this low since my chemo/transplant days. Fever, chills, aches, night-sweats. It gets bad enough on Thursday morning that I ask Susan to call the doctor. He confirms I have pneumonia and puts me on antibiotics.

I need to get better in time for surgery on September 2 to take out some lymph nodes in my neck and probably one of my parotid glands. I will meet with a radiation oncologist this week to see if that's an alternative to surgery but I'm no fan of radiation either.

Dr. John Cichon will be doing the cutting. He trained at the Mayo Clinic. Here's what their site says about a parotidectomy:

The parotid glands are the body's largest salivary glands. Located in front of the ears, the parotid glands extend to the area beneath the earlobe along the lower border of the jawbone. About 80 percent of salivary gland tumors are found in the parotid gland. Only about 20 percent of parotid gland tumors are malignant. [Lucky me!]

The surgery can be complicated because a nerve controlling facial movement runs through the gland. Mayo specialists do not recommend the removal of just the parotid tumor (lumpectomy) because microscopic tumor cells can remain in the wound, causing the tumor to recur. What also passes through the parotid gland besides the facial nerve are the external carotid artery and the retromandibular vein, which is why I want a steady hand on the scalpel.

The procedure will include doing biopsies of surrounding tissue to look for the origin of the cancer and making sure it isn't traveling along the major nerves. If it is, they will be removed.

Five Insights

The fact that I've got another cancer is overwhelming but not unusual given the nature of the disease. From my experience and research I've gleaned the following insights:

1. *Cancer is an accumulation of accidental cellular events* that conspire to take down the whole system, slowly building momentum over the years until it reaches a tipping point and then cascades out of control toward the grave.

2. *Cancer can take decades to mature*, during which the initial mutation is augmented by other random genetic changes, fueled by carcinogens in our food and environment and super-charged by stress.

3. *Cancer is born in, and borne along by, the genes*, as Dr. Mukherjee points out: "Abnormal genes governed all aspects of cancer's behavior. Cascades of aberrant signals, originating in mutated genes, fanned out within the cancer cell, promoting survival, accelerating growth, enabling mobility, recruiting blood

vessels, enhancing nourishment, drawing oxygen—sustaining cancer's life."

4. *Cancer hijacks the body's normal processes to its own narcissistic ends.* There's nothing extraneous about cancer. It doesn't invent new proteins or pathways but exploits existing ones, like mitosis and motility, while overriding built-in safeguards like apoptosis and tumor-suppressor genes.

5. *Cancer has vulnerabilities; it can be beaten*—or at least beaten back for several years—by a combination of healthy habits and medical treatments. My seven-fold strategy includes a positive attitude, a sense of humor, a plant-based diet, targeted intervention (surgery, radiation, chemotherapy), submissive prayer, a focus on others and the loving support of family and friends.

The last point is the most important for the millions with cancer and the countless others who love and support us.

One Good Thing About Cancer

Cancer is a very unsocial disease, being neither contagious nor infectious. (Diseases spread by direct contact are contagious; those spread through air or water are infectious.) Researchers, oncologists, nurses, caregivers or family never "catch" cancer, no matter how intimate their involvement with its victims.

Cancer is a micro-evolutionary process that works on the cellular level, as explained by biologist David Sloan Wilson:

Cell division is exceptionally well supervised. A new copy of DNA is made, like a monk transcribing holy text. The copy is proofread and corrected with such accuracy that the final error rate can be less than one in a million for any given letter of the text. Still, the entire text contains millions of letters, so most copies include a few errors. Many mutations have no effect on the cell's function. Most of those that do are quickly detected and destroyed by the immune system.

In the case of cancer, enough mutants survive and adapt to cause havoc. Over many years and through thousands of iterations they morph and multiply until they destroy their host.

Every mutational "advance" that enables the cell line to avoid its "predators" (immune system), beat its "competitors" (the normally functioning cells), and colonize other areas of the body (metastasis) brings it closer to its own demise. Even if a tumor remains benign, it will wink out of existence with the natural death of the organism, lacking any mechanism for getting from one body to another.

Did you catch the glint of good news in that last sentence? For all its stubborn ferocity, cancer is myopic—and sterile.

o   o   o

"Down to their innate molecular core,
cancer cells are hyperactive, survival-endowed,
scrappy, fecund, inventive copies of ourselves."
— Dr. Siddhartha Mukherjee

NECK DISSECTION

A "neck dissection" is what Dr. Cichon calls my procedure in the operating room. In post-op I tell him he needs to change his terminology. Dissection is what you do to frogs in high school biology, and it doesn't work out so well for the frogs. I should know; I was the top biology student at Sheridan High School, class of 1970. That was back when textbooks were in black and white and Coke came in cans, not grams.

My seventh surgery in the last three years took more than six hours. Coming out of the amnesia after that long is a very unpleasant experience. Dr. Cichon and his team removed my parotid gland, some nodes and surrounding tissue, including a small piece of my ear lobe. There was enough skin to pull the edges together. Wonderful stuff the epidermis; amazing what can be done with it. There shouldn't be much lasting damage from the operation, either in looks or in function.

The margins were clear, the doc tells me, which means he believes he got all the cancer. But he still can't tell what kind of cancer it is. Perhaps not squamous as originally suspected. Maybe a more virulent form of lymphoma. That would not be good news. We'll see what the pathologist finds and go from there.

The people I have met in the medical profession over the years have been wonderful and the care usually top notch. But if you're in the system often enough you're bound to catch an off night. When I get to the surgical floor I have to ask for my gown to be changed from the one I had on during the operation. My bedding wasn't changed after the operation, perhaps because I was only going to be there one night. I finally have to ask for a new blanket because the blood smear grosses me out. The pillowcase and bottom sheet are likewise stained but it seems too much hassle to change them.

I was told I would be allowed to sleep between having my vitals checked at midnight and 4 a.m. but I know better. The gentleman in the bed next to me is checked hourly, with conversation and lights, the latter usually left on. His machine beeps because of a low battery until a nurse finally changes it.

The pharmacy won't give me the sleeping pill the doctor had specifically requested but sends up a generic pill. I know from experience it won't work, which is why I had the doctor specify something that would. No go with the pharmacist; rules are rules, especially at 10 p.m. The nurse finally has to walk to the pharmacy with a handwritten note saying "patient refuses substitution." And I'll have a fight with insurance down the road over that one pill, which ends up not working either.

There's nothing like a night awake in a hospital bed, getting reacquainted with your body, trying to "feel" where the pieces are missing. I can't. I have a small bowl over my left ear and two rubber bulbs the size of racquetballs hanging from drains in my neck. I can see blood collecting in each, which is a good sign.

Pathology Report

My post-surgical pathology report shows:

» High-grade (fast-growing) squamous cell carcinoma in the parotid gland and some surrounding nerves and muscle. Rare.

» The edges were clean, which is an indication the surgeon got all the tumor. Good.

» The fifteen lymph nodes that were removed showed no signs of cancer. Very Good.

Squamous cell carcinoma is the lesser of two evils. If the lymphoma had returned that would mean it was resistant to the chemo and that my bone marrow transplant had failed. Squamous cell is a skin cancer that had to start somewhere other than the parotid gland and lymph nodes but we don't know where. It could show up elsewhere as mysteriously as it did in my neck and face, including in a vital organ.

The overall outcome is positive but the battle continues and I have to get my head around that. I will learn more about what's going on and what my treatment options are when Dr. Dax goes over the pathology report with me. I assume he'll recommend radiation to kill any cancer cells that may be in the nerves. (This could be why I felt numbness before there was a tumor.)

I'm not a big fan of radiation and have to do more research before making my decision. What it destroys will be permanently gone. I could take a "wait and see" approach, but if there are still some tumor cells and the cancer returns, radiation won't be as effective.

Despite the gnarly scar, the pain is minimal due to the cut nerves. The left side of my mouth doesn't work like it used to, causing some issues with eating. I also can't sleep on my left side unless I rest just the top of my head on the edge of the pillow and put another pillow under my chest so there's no weight on my cheek or ear.

Susan and I have talked more since the surgery about what happens if cancer gets the upper hand. We agree that we want to be proactive in preparing for the future. We don't have a lot to work with but the goal is to get ourselves (or Susan) set up in a sustainable long-term situation. Without being too morbid, we've also brought up the subject with the kids. Whatever comes, we will deal with it openly as a family. Being able to do so is a great blessing.

o　o　o

"Nothing that is worth doing can be achieved in our lifetime,
therefore we must be saved by hope.
Nothing which is true or beautiful or good
makes complete sense in any immediate context of history,
therefore we must be saved by faith.
Nothing we do, however virtuous, can be accomplished alone,
therefore we must be saved by love."
—Reinhold Neibur

RECLINER REFLECTIONS

Susan brings me home on Saturday morning, September 6, and I lie around all day with a few walks on the treadmill. My first night at home is a trial. I feel like I'm hallucinating part of the time because I'm seeing and responding to strange things. I find my way back to my faithful recliner around 5 a.m. I'm restless and having problems keeping my throat clear, the left side of which doesn't work too well.

Slow recovery day on Monday. I get a little reading and writing done and take a few short walks. I pop a sleeping pill at night that keeps me out until about 4:30; then it's over to the recliner to count breaths and swallows until dawn. I'm thankful there's not much pain, just the problem of drainage and the feeling of being partially choked. The stitches span a good eight inches; we'll see what kind of scar I get as a souvenir.

The nights are the worst. They just have to be endured, one long minute after the next. I talk to God during these quiet hours. I have thoughts about him and a few insights but no sense that he's physically present—if I can use that phrase of an immaterial being whose center is everywhere and circumference is nowhere. If I want to talk to Susan, I can call her and she will come and sit with me. I can call Andy or Scotty on the phone and have a two-way conversation, but I can't manage to do either of these with Jesus.

I also think about my future. If my cancer returns I would have to consider radiation and perhaps a donor bone marrow transplant. I'm hesitant to do the first and very reluctant to consider the second given the reduced quality of life afterward. My first choice is to pursue other treatment options: integrated medicine, alternative therapies, diet and lifestyle changes.

I reflect on conversations with family and friends. The shadow of my death hung ominously over each. One friend asked how long I expected to live and I told him I'm ambivalent because while I feel okay from day to day, I know I'm on my third bout of cancer and the latest one is high-grade and treatment resistant.

In retrospect I can't really settle for ambivalent. I have to work hard at staying alive because there are people and experiences worth living for. I know I can't will or work myself to complete wellness but I can tilt the odds in my favor with some concerted effort. For starters, I determine to increase my exercise routine, fine-tune my diet and plug into some of the cancer groups to see how I can help others.

I want to make the most of whatever time I have left. I want to keep writing about my experiences and insights. I think of how books have enriched my own life and connected me to my fellow pilgrims and I want to be a part of that honorable tradition.

Living Between Shoes

"Waiting for the other shoe to drop" is a cliché that means, "waiting for a related announcement or event to occur after an initial announcement or situation. When waiting for the other shoe to drop, one expects a pending situation to occur that is dependent upon an initial event."

Living with cancer is living between shoes.

After my first chemo regimen—six rounds in four months—I had three clear scans. I got a cancer survivor certificate from my oncologist, a party from my family and the obligatory T-shirt that said, "I Beat Cancer and All I Got Was This Lousy T-Shirt!" But cancer is one badass disease that doesn't like to be taunted. A few months later the lymphoma returned, which meant more intense chemo and a bone marrow transplant.

The lymphoma stays at bay but squamous cell carcinoma comes a-callin' a year later. The wrestling match continues.

The specter of cancer casts a shadow but not a cloud for me. It puts life in perspective but not morbidly so. It helps me savor the mundane and be more present in the moment. It makes me more thankful for the gifts bestowed by everyday providence.

I vacillate between "Providence" and "providence," not sure how much to ascribe to divine intervention. God is the author of all *possibilities*, but as to specifics, if we give him credit for blessings—surviving cancer—what about holding him accountable for allowing the cancer in the first place? These are two sides of the same coin, one that religious people don't flip very often.

We praise God for healing but are at a loss to explain why others who pray just as fervently don't make it. It's as if an all-knowing doctor decides to save some people while refusing to help others who are just as needy. How would such a physician be treated by his community? Hailed for his compassion, albeit limited, or excoriated for not doing more?

Most religions try to explain this enigma. Some do a more coherent job than others but all rely on a fair amount of interpretative speculation. We know less than we claim. One thing we do know is that everyone dies. The other shoe always drops—sometimes unexpectedly fast as in an auto crash; sometimes excruciatingly slow as with cancer. Each way has its pluses and minuses—not that we get to choose.

What we get to choose is how to live between shoes.

o   o   o

"There is a reason why God limits our days."
"Why?"
"To make each one precious."
—*The Time Keeper*, Mitch Albom

SHOT IN THE FACE

More than half the people being treated for cancer in the United States undergo radiation and on Monday, September 20, I will join their ranks. While my surgery successfully removed the tumor, there was some indication the cancer might be tracking along a nerve. If microscopic cancer cells are left behind, they could start growing again.

I was reluctant to undergo radiation but my research has convinced me to proceed. Squamous cell is a treatment-resistant carcinoma so I need all the available tools to fight it. The particular type of radiation I will be getting is called TomoTherapy. This therapeutic radiation uses high-energy beams of photons or charged particles to damage the DNA of cancer cells so they can't reproduce.

TomoTherapy is a form of Intensity Modulated Radiation Therapy (IMRT) that delivers said radiation slice-by-slice. (Tomo is Greek for "slice.") This approach has some real advantages, according to tomotherapy.com:

> 360° delivery. The TomoTherapy Hi Art treatment system's linear accelerator is mounted to a CT scanner-like ring gantry, which means TomoTherapy treatments can be delivered continuously, from all angles around the patient. More beam

directions give physicians more control in how they plan treatments—and more assurance that dose will be confined to the tumor, reducing the risk of short-and long-term side effects.

The TomoTherapy treatment system uses a patented multi-leaf collimator that divides the radiation beam into beamlets, all aimed at the tumor. Typically, tens of thousands of beamlets are used in a single TomoTherapy treatment session. Powerful software optimizes the contribution of each one to the total tumor dose, minimizing exposure to healthy tissue.

This makes TomoTherapy sound like an expensive spa treatment. Who wouldn't want to be gently massaged by thousands of soothing beamlets of energy?

Me!

The hardest thing to wrap my mind around is the number of treatments—thirty-three! I have to go in Monday through Friday for almost seven weeks. The sessions only last fifteen minutes but the effects are cumulative. Side effects include:

» fatigue
» skin damage, hair loss
» dry mouth, painful swallowing, loss of taste
» possible atherosclerosis of blood vessels
» staying alive

Unlike chemotherapy, what radiation kills stays dead, which is one reason for my reluctance. Radiation is another of those experiences not on my bucket list but here it is, demanding face time (sic). At least the ability to target a specific area and minimize peripheral damage is fairly good with TomoTherapy.

How is my psyche doing with this latest challenge? I'm adjusting. The process started last Friday with the making of a cast for me to lie in. This ensures I'll be in the same position for every treatment. A mask was also made to hold my head still while I get shot in the face and neck with high energy particle beams.

TomoTherapy radiation requires the victim, er, I mean patient, to lie perfectly still for about fifteen minutes. To achieve this, a body mold is cast from the waist up. The hostage, er, I mean patient, is put in this mold for each treatment. For head and neck radiation, the head must be completely immobilized. A form-fitting mask is cast for each mark, er, I mean, patient and clamped down to the table, which is then pulled into the CT/radiation machine.

This experience is not for the claustrophobic. Fortunately it is painless at the time and the side effects aren't felt by the patsy, er, I mean patient, until later in the cycle, which in my case will last for thirty-three treatments. Eventually the weightless photons will do substantial damage to the interior of my cells—the normal as well as the cancerous ones.

I wonder if they'll let me take my mask home for Halloween.

Going Platinum

You can go platinum by either selling ten million albums or by having the stuff injected directly into your veins, which is the route I'm taking.

I just finished my twenty-third round of chemo (September 27). I should have a chair named after me in the clinic. I've tried to talk the nurses into a Rewards Card for frequent customers. Something like every tenth treatment being free. As much as these pharmaceuticals cost, that would be a five-figure savings.

The drug of choice for this round of chemo is cisplatin, which is a form of platinum. Why put a cancer-causing poison into the body to fight cancer? One word: apoptosis. Apoptosis is "a normal, genetically regulated process leading to the death of cells triggered by the presence or absence of certain stimuli, such as DNA damage.

This is also called "programmed cell death."

Between fifty and seventy billion cells die daily due to apoptosis in the average healthy adult. Cells that ignore their genetic instructions and refuse to die result in potentially terminal diseases like cancer.

Cisplatin causes cross-linking that damages the RNA or DNA, which causes apoptosis in cancer cells. It may also interfere with the proteins that carry signals back and forth from the nucleus to the membrane. Cisplatin is given in lower doses along with radiation to administer a one-two punch to stubborn cancers.

But cisplatin also encourages apoptosis in healthy cells, hence the side effects, according to chemocare.com:

Chemotherapy is most effective at killing cells that are rapidly dividing. Unfortunately, chemotherapy does not know the difference between the cancerous cells and the normal cells. The normal cells will grow back and be healthy but in the meantime, side effects occur. The cells most commonly affected are the blood cells, the cells in the mouth, stomach and bowel, and the hair follicles.

My previous chemo regimes were not pleasant, and this cycle is swiftly headed that direction. My energy level is down and I'm nauseated most of the day. I don't know how bad it would be without the meds I'm taking but I don't want to find out. Pretty soon the mouth sores, hair loss and other side effects will kick in. Thankfully, the radiation treatments at this stage are painless.

It doesn't help that I haven't been able to find work the last two months or that I haven't been paid for a job I did in July. I can't pay the bills and am going further into debt to cover the mortgage and keep the lights on. My debt-to-income ratio is too high to refinance the house so I can't get any relief that way.

Still, I'm alive and thankful to be so. I was sitting on the edge of the bed this morning and thinking about another day of subpar health. I've been living under a shadow for more than three years and I wouldn't have missed any of it despite the pain and suffering. I've seen four children added to the Hamel clan and have had some wonderful experiences with their parents—my kids. I've enjoyed my friends and written more words that may someday be read by curious readers. I haven't done nearly everything I wanted to, but I've done a whole lot more than if I were dead!

○   ○   ○

"Cancer therapy is like beating the dog with a stick
to get rid of his fleas."
—Anna Deavere Smith

NOUN *AND* VERB

Dictionaries list "cancer" as a noun (person, place or thing), but it should also be defined as a verb (expressing action, state, or a relation between things). Cancer produces things like tumors, but at the core it's an aggressive, self-generating action. "We misunderstand cancer by making it a noun," insists Dr. David Agus. "I like to tell people that cancer isn't so much something that you 'get' or 'have' as it's something that the body does. ... Instead of saying, 'Somebody has cancer,' we should say, 'They are cancering.'"

"Cancering" is a regular part of life and our bodies usually manage to keep it in check. But over the years—and for a variety of reasons—the balance can incrementally shift until a lethal tipping point is reached and we are diagnosed with cancer.

Cancering is not an invasion; it's a mutiny. There are no foreign attackers or outside contagions. Our own cells are mutating and multiplying out of control. These rebels put their individual survival above the survival of the whole body.

Cancering is "civil war"—an oxymoron if there ever was one.

Those of us whose cancering is out of control have a pretty good idea what will kill us—if not soon, eventually. Cancer can go into remission but it seldom gives up. (Despite billions spent on research, the death rate for cancer dropped only five percent from

1950 to 2005.) We suspect it's hiding in the genes, biding its time. Want to know what else people with cancer think but might not verbalize?

» Feel free to share the miracle cure that saved your second cousin's brother-in-law but don't push it. We've heard everything from cottage cheese and flaxseed diets to coffee enemas. (I'm not an MD but I'm pretty sure that's not where coffee goes.)

» It's wonderful to be loved but we don't always want to be the center of attention. If we're in the hospital or recovering at home, check to see if we're up for visitors before coming by.

» Don't make it your mission to lift our spirits. It's not easy being optimistic some days.

» We don't need you to explain what God is doing through the cancer.

» Sometimes we hardly recognize the person in the mirror. We worry you won't remember the healthy, vital people we were for most of our lives but the sick and feeble shells cancer has reduced us to.

» Caregivers need care too. Think about doing something special for our spouses or families.

The Best People

While in the waiting room before my radiation treatment on October 3, I pick up a copy of *Colorado Springs Style* magazine. The cover story is about the best doctors in town and my oncologist (Dax Kurbegov) and radiation oncologist (Mark Hazuka) are both featured, as is the surgeon who did my port surgeries (Larry Dillon). It's wonderful to be in such capable hands.

My experience with physicians has been much better than Voltaire's, who wrote, "Doctors are men who prescribe medicines of which they know little, to cure diseases of which they know less, in human beings of whom they know nothing."

When I asked Dax for a short blurb for this book, he wrote a whole page. Not because he has a ton of time for such things but because he has a lot of passion for what he does. Here's part of what he said:

> CANCER. It's the big "C" word. We speak of it in whispers, eyes downcast. We're afraid to probe too deeply into our family histories lest we somehow invite cancer into our lives by the simple act of discovering another family member's cancer journey. Though most of us know little of what cancer is or how it affects our bodies, we certainly know enough not to want it.
>
> I'm a cancer doc, a medical oncologist. No one wants to meet me … at least professionally. My life's work revolves around shepherding heroic men and women through their cancer journeys. It involves deconstructing societal perceptions of what it means to be a victim of cancer. It involves replacing ignorance with understanding. It involves transforming the victim into an empowered survivor.

Most of us have great difficulty facing the Grim Reaper once; imagine a vocation where he's your daily sparring partner! That's an emotional burden few can shoulder. I've come to have a deep respect for those who choose oncology as a profession. Their commitment is one reason I'm still alive.

I've found the same quality of people throughout the Memorial Health System, from receptionists and social workers to nurses and technicians. They are highly competent and genuinely concerned professionals, which I greatly appreciate since they are helping to keep me around.

My all-time champion caregiver is Susan. She has been a

lifesaver for me and countless others over the years. I was reminded of this at the recent Life Network Gala. Susan has been working there for fifteen years and has been the Director of the Pregnancy Center since 2002. This past year the Center helped almost 8,000 clients and, as a result, 251 babies were born who otherwise might not be alive today.

I am so proud of Susan and the work she does every day. She's uniquely called and gifted to help people in crisis—especially her husband.

Long Days, Longer Nights

Being sick is a full-time job. I wind up spending seven hours at the cancer clinic in a combination of doctor visit, chemo and radiation. Then I spend another hour at the pharmacist picking up the prescriptions.

My overwhelming feeling at the end of the day is gratitude: gratitude to God that I'm still alive; gratitude to the medical personnel who take care of me so compassionately; gratitude for a health system that has spent hundreds of thousands of dollars on my care; gratitude for family and friends who support and pray for me—the list goes on. There are many things to be discouraged and overwhelmed by, but I choose to see the encouraging and positive parts of the picture—at least for today.

I can't recall the last time I slept through the night, and I don't have young children. Even Michael-Jackson-strength prescription drugs don't help. My cancer, bone marrow transplant, auto accident and surgeries have recalibrated my circadian rhythms. I didn't choose these calamities but I get to choose how I respond. Here are three things I do:

Talk to myself: Most days it's difficult to have a decent internal dialogue. Too many interruptions; too much background noise. Volleying an idea between cerebral hemispheres is harder than sustaining a rally against Rafael Nadal. But in the dark I can leisurely bounce it off the wall like Steve McQueen in *The Great Escape* until I catch something I can use.

Listen for God: I say listen *for* God, not listen *to* God, because I haven't heard another voice in the nocturnal silence. I have thoughts I assign to God or assume he's prompted but it's not a two-way conversation. Still, I listen—and I remind God I'm listening—because I believe he speaks and I'm hopeful he will do so to me one of these nights.

Pilot my dreams: When I sleep, my dreams are on autopilot. If I'm semi-awake, I can slip a hand onto the controls. In this ethereal landscape I can ride the thermals like a glider. The currents rule the air but I can make some tweaks to better enjoy the scenery.

My advice for insomniacs: Do something about your night musings the next day. Write down the insight, act on the idea, answer neglected email, call the creditor, do lunch, clean up your in-box, back off at work, speak up at church, get with the person who needs to hear you say, "I'm sorry," or "I forgive you."

Make the most of these golden hours; they are precious, if sometimes unwanted, gifts.

o o o

"If you woke up breathing, congratulations!
You have another chance!"
—Andrea Boydston

DRINKING DOWNRIVER

No chemo yesterday (November 1) or last Monday for that matter. I was all hooked up but they wouldn't give me the juice. My blood counts were too low, particularly my platelets. The normal range is 150-450. I'm down to forty-nine. My white blood cells are down to two and my reds are also below normal.

Not surprising; I've been on the decline since starting on cisplatin. It affects the bone marrow where blood cells are made and my marrow doesn't recover as fast as it did before my transplant. This means I'm only getting two-thirds of the chemo I'm supposed to during radiation, which may slightly reduce its overall effectiveness.

In his epic history of cancer, *The Emperor of All Maladies*, Dr. Siddhartha Mukherjee recounts the introduction of cisplatin in the 1970s:

> The drug provided an unremitting nausea, a queasiness of such penetrating force and quality that had rarely been encountered in the history of medicine: on average, patients treated with the drug vomited twelve times a day. In the 1970s, there were few antinausea drugs. Most patients had to be given intravenous fluids to tide them through. ... In nursing slang, the drug came to be known as "Cisflatten."

189

The side effects, however revolting, were considered minor dues to pay (probably not by the patients) for an otherwise miraculous drug. Cisplatin was touted as the epic chemotherapeutic product of the late 1970s; the quintessential example of how curing cancer involved pushing patients nearly to the brink of death. By 1978, cisplatin-based chemotherapy was the new vogue in cancer pharmacology; every conceivable combination was being tested on thousands of patients across America.

Cisplatin is still a frontline chemo drug thirty-five years later. When I asked my oncologist why he was treating me with such an old medicine he said, "Because we haven't found anything more toxic." At least the anti-nausea meds are better. And fortunately for me, I got a reduced dose to augment the radiation, not the full measure many patients have to endure.

The aftereffects of chemo are like "drinking downriver from the herd," as Kinky Friedman would say. There's a lot of crap involved.

Chemo leaves a bad taste in the mouth that feels like a filmy coating of dead cells. Nothing tastes good. Dry mouth from radiation doesn't help. My stomach is usually queasy and doesn't appreciate visitors, which is why I'm down to 143 pounds. Then there's the fatigue and sleep deprivation.

Chemo is done for now and radiation ends Wednesday. My CBC (complete blood count) shows no improvement and my white cells continue to decline; it will take time to climb back into the normal range. (I know; since when have I been normal?)

I'm looking forward to the holidays and am very thankful for the treatment I've received and the wonderful people who walked me through it. It wasn't pleasant but drinking downriver is a small price to pay for staying topside a while longer.

Sixty-six Gray

Wednesday, November 9, was the last of my radiation treatments for HNSCC (head/neck squamous cell carcinoma). I got a call in the morning saying the machine had broken down and to come in the afternoon. Anything to drag this out. But now I can retire my mask and mold.

In the last seven weeks I've received sixty-six Gy (gray) of radiation in thirty-three doses of two Gy each. Wikipedia defines gray:

> One gray is the absorption of one joule of energy, in the form of ionizing radiation, divided by one kilogram of matter. ... The gray measures the deposited energy of radiation. The biological effects vary by the type and energy of the radiation and the organism and tissues involved. ...
>
> A whole-body exposure to 5 or more gray of high-energy radiation at one time usually leads to death within 14 days. This dosage represents 375 joules for a 75 kg adult. [This is why the dose is divided into multiple treatments.] Since gray are such large amounts of radiation, medical use of radiation is typically measured in milligray (mGy). ...
>
> The salivary glands and tear glands have a radiation tolerance of about 30 Gy in 2 Gy fractions, a dose which is exceeded by most radical head and neck cancer treatments, potentially causing dryness. Dry mouth (xerostomia) and dry eyes (xerophthalmia) can become irritating long-term problems and severely reduce the patient's quality of life.

I'm pretty dry now but shouldn't have long-term problems because of the 360-degree approach of TomoTherapy. At least that's the theory. Too bad I can't blame my dry sense of humor or mental problems on radiation but the beamlets were aimed so as only to pass through the lower part of the brain.

o   o   o

"Chemotherapy isn't good for you.
So when you feel bad, as I am feeling now, you think,
'Well that's a good thing because it's supposed to be poison.'
If it's making the tumor feel this queasy, then I'm OK with it."
—Christopher Hitchens

CONVALESCENCE

It's been four weeks since my last chemo and almost a week since my last radiation and my appetite is worse than ever. Just the thought of food makes my stomach queasy. I force myself to eat but it's not a pleasant experience. Things that I think will taste good don't, once I stick them in my mouth.

If this is the result of a lesser dose of cisplatin, I don't want to ever try a full dose. Perhaps it's the cumulative effect of everything my body has been through but it's not recovering very well this time.

It would be nice to have my taste buds back by Thanksgiving.

I'm finally sleeping without the aid of pharmaceuticals for the first time in months. I'm even staying asleep long enough to make it through the entire cycle a few times. According to WebMD.com,

> Sleep is prompted by natural cycles of activity in the brain and consists of two basic states: rapid eye movement (REM) sleep and non-rapid eye movement (NREM) sleep, which consists of Stages 1 through 4. ... A completed cycle of sleep consists of a progression from stages 1-4 before REM sleep is attained, then the cycle starts over again.

The benefits of REM sleep can be felt the next day, as explained by Helpguide.org:

> During REM sleep, your brain consolidates and processes the information you've learned during the day, forms neural connections that strengthen memory, and replenishes its supply of neurotransmitters, including feel-good chemicals such as serotonin and dopamine that boost your mood during the day.

It's "invigorating" to wake up remembering bits and pieces of dreams. That's not a word I've been able to use much in the past few years.

Resurrecting Patients
I didn't realize until reading Dr. Mukherjee's book the link between chemo and bone marrow transplants. Transplants have been a front-line treatment for some cancers since the middle of the last century. I had mine in June of 2009 after my NHL failed to respond to chemotherapy. The procedure was originally conceived of as a way to resurrect cancer patients after administering "blisteringly" high doses of chemo, as Dr. Mukherjee recounts:

> The dose limit of a drug is set by its toxicity to normal cells. For most chemotherapy drugs, that dose limit rested principally on a single organ—the bone marrow. ... The bone marrow represented the frontier of toxicity, an unbreakable barrier that limited the capacity to deliver obliterative chemotherapy—the "red ceiling" as some oncologists called it.

Bone marrow transplants made it possible to give five-to-ten times the lethal dose of drugs. But rebooting patients with fresh marrow didn't initially work. One trial with leukemia patients in the 1980s had an eighty-eight percent fatality rate! And the twelve "survivors" didn't last very long.

Transplants produce a host of complications, from graft-versus-host disease (GVHD) to secondary solid-tumor cancers, but outcomes have steadily improved over the decades. I've had a second cancer—squamous cell carcinoma—as a result of having my red ceiling reconstructed. The internal remodel hasn't been pleasant but it's given me two-and-a-half more years of life, for which I'm very thankful.

My transplant also connected me to a worldwide community of sufferers, survivors, family members, caregivers, researchers, doctors, nurses and countless other concerned souls. Including, it turns out, lawyers. As I mentioned earlier, the year after my transplant the Institute for Justice contacted me regarding an effort to change the laws governing bone marrow transplants.

Cancer can isolate us as we focus on staying alive. But it can also connect us to others in a common battle for survival. Helping others is actually one of the healthiest things we can do for ourselves.

○   ○   ○

"Here is the test to find whether your mission
on earth is finished.
If you're alive, it isn't."
—Richard Bach

UNHAPPY THANKSGIVING

On Thanksgiving Day, Susan and I enjoyed our protein shakes and some casual kitchen conversation before driving to Denver for family dinner at our son Nate and daughter-in-law Jenn's home. Susan's sister Ruth rode with us and we were all in a relaxed mood.

Susan had gone through a rough patch at work but was now on vacation. We were flying to Phoenix in a few days to spend time with her sister Janet and husband Bruce for some much-needed rest. I had completed my radiation and chemo treatments and was slowly regaining strength.

At Nate's I busied myself in the kitchen while Susan went off to see the grandkids, including the newest addition to the Hamel clan, Eli David Briggs. After several minutes, I called her to help me but got no response. Then Ruth said she'd heard a noise in the guest bathroom but assumed it was one of the kids. I checked the door and found it locked. There was no response to my banging. I grabbed the key from above the door knowing what I would find inside.

Before the paramedics arrived, Nate (a Denver firefighter) gave his mom CPR, not something a son ever expects to have to do. The medics kept it up all the way to the hospital but Susan never regained consciousness. Cause of death: acute heart failure.

About two hundred sixty-seven thousand women die annually from heart disease, six times more than will succumb to breast cancer. Dr. Richard Fleming notes, "Half the people who have heart disease find out they have a heart problem by dropping dead. That's the first symptom they have."

What painful irony. After all she did to keep me alive, Susan was the one to die first. Losing my life-partner of thirty-seven years has been the hardest thing I've had to endure by far.

Celebration Service

We held Susan's Celebration Service on a stormy Saturday (December 3) at Vanguard Church. More than five hundred people made it through the snow to be with us. Our four children all shared movingly about their mother. I managed to make it through the eulogy I wrote without breaking down. In part, I said:

> I'm currently writing a book called, *We Will Be Landing Shortly: Now What?* Susie's death on Thanksgiving Day is a solemn reminder that we all are on "final approach." Some of us will have time to get our seatbacks and tray tables in the upright and locked position. Others will crash with little warning and no time to prepare. The one invariable is that every one of us will be landing shortly.
>
> Susan was ready because of how she lived her life every day, in public and in private. I just wasn't ready to say goodbye so soon. Her legacy is her family and the thousands of people she blessed over the years.
>
> She always had open arms, a listening ear, a non-judgmental heart, an accepting nature, an inviting smile, a steadfast faith and treats for her grandkids.
>
> Susan wasn't perfect. She never got the hang of gossip; didn't know how to carry a grudge; couldn't keep her checkbook

closed when it came to others, would accept just about anybody as a friend; and routinely welcomed strangers into our home for months at a time.

I know where Susan is today and I'm happy for her and at peace. I expect to join her some day. Maybe then she can explain to me what in the world God was thinking when he left me without adult supervision—and why he let her cut in line in front of me.

Susie, you can never be replaced, and you will never be forgotten. I love you deeply. Always have; always will.

o   o   o

"Death leaves a heartache no one can heal,
love leaves a memory no one can steal."
—Irish tombstone

SNEAK ATTACK

I traveled to Phoenix the last week in December with a cough that incubated into pneumonia. I spent six hours in the Chandler Regional Medical Center ER on Wednesday (January 4) and was called back on Thursday when a culture revealed the infection had spread to the blood. Turns out I had *streptococcus pneumoniae,* or "strep-pneumonia." I didn't know there was such a hybrid, but trust me to get the weird version of a typical disease. And trust me to get it in a place where my insurance company doesn't operate.

Strep-pneumonia is dangerous and I'm thankful the ER staff caught it. I'm getting a bag-o-biotics as I type this and hope to be released with pills at some point to enjoy the rest of my Phoenix stay. Always the optimist. But this time around the infection spread to my blood and posed a real threat to other organs, hence the hospitalization. It might be that each time I get sick it's more serious because of my weakened immune system. I have to learn to be more careful about germs.

There are more than fifty types of pneumonia, which is basically fluid and/or swelling in the lungs. It can be caused by fungus, bacteria or a virus. If it's on both sides of the lungs, it's double pneumonia. Mine is double—of course.

Pneumonia is nothing to sneeze at. According to Medicine.Net:

> Prior to the discovery of antibiotics, one-third of all people who developed pneumonia subsequently died from the infection. Currently, over 3 million people develop pneumonia each year in the United States. Over a half a million of these people are admitted to a hospital for treatment. Although most of these people recover, approximately 5% will die from pneumonia. Pneumonia is the sixth leading cause of death in the United States.

Famous people who died of pneumonia include Fred Astaire, James Brown (godfather of soul, not the football player), René Descartes, Bob Hope, Lawrence Welk, Leo Tolstoy, Geronimo, General Norman Schwarzkopf and Oral Roberts. (Being inveterately curious, I look up such things.)

I remember the weakness and tiredness from when I had pneumonia last August but I didn't have as much chest pain then. It feels like a cracked rib but the doctor diagnoses it as *pleurisy*, which the Mayo Clinic says, "occurs when the double membrane (pleura) that lines the inside of your chest cavity and surrounds each of your lungs becomes inflamed. Also called pleuritis, pleurisy typically causes sharp pain, almost always when inhaling and exhaling."

At least it only hurts when I inhale or exhale. The pain isn't too bad during the day but when it stabs me awake at night, it's excruciating.

The love and support of family and friends has been fantastic. My hosts, Dave and Debbie Briggs, have been amazing in going above and beyond the call of hospitality. I've learned a valuable lesson from this sneak attack in my warfare with germs. Next time I will travel under an assumed name so I can't be so easily tracked by ill fortune.

I've also learned that what doesn't kill you—can still make you pretty miserable.

It's been great having Julie and Eli here with me. We've enjoyed some wonderful talks and walks—special times. I thoroughly enjoy all my kids and grandkids. They are a healing tonic and help me keep life in perspective. They remind me why it's worth sticking around as long as I can.

I finally get some good news on the health front a few weeks after returning home from Phoenix. My scan on Monday (January 23) comes back clean. September's surgery appears to have been successful in that there is no sign of cancer in my neck or anywhere else. I have some persistent pneumonia loitering about but it's a good day for me when the doc can only find pneumonia and not something worse.

A friend and fellow cancer survivor had surgery on his neck the same day I got my scan results. They removed a cancerous tumor, which means his battle continues without reprieve. Why am I clean this time around and he isn't? Add this to the bazillion "why" questions that don't have answers. The question we can answer, regardless of whether we are clean or cancerous is, "What are we going to do about it?"

Homo Infirmitus

Science divides humanity into various hominid species including:

Homo Habilis – "handy man," user of tools

Homo Erectus – "to put up, set upright"

Homo Sapien – "knowing man"

Let me suggest another:

Homo Infirmitus – "weakness, ailment"

From minor aches to terminal diseases, infirmities are part of being finite. Is there an intrinsic reason why this has to be? We are indeed "fearfully and wonderfully made," but why were we created with all these design flaws?

Every religion and philosophy has an explanation for suffering. Judeo-Christianity ascribes it to sin. A moral choice is said to have triggered physical decay, doing to the body what fermentation does to the grape—set it to rotting.

Humans have an innate sense that something's wrong; this isn't how it's supposed to be. Hence the almost universal belief in an afterlife where we will be fixed. Pain will be eliminated and pleasure will be maximized or the locus of both—the body—radically upgraded or jettisoned altogether. In the mean time our theology helps us cope by giving meaning to the madness. Christians believe the incarnation is God undertaking our rescue. But even he can't avoid the price of admission into the game of life—suffering and death.

As if enduring our own pain weren't enough, we can experience the pain of others. The emotional connection to those we love is a nerve bundle through which we enjoy the most exquisite ecstasies and agonies.

Pain and suffering take up far too much of life if you ask me. But then, nobody asked me.

o   o   o

"We are born wet, naked, and hungry.
Then things get worse."
—Author Unknown

MEDITATE ON THIS

Meditation can be a vital part of dealing with cancer. Dr. Servan-Schreiber touted the practice in the best cancer book I've read, *AntiCancer: A New Way of Life*. He noted that when breast and prostate cancer patients in a Calgary University study began meditating, "Their white blood cells, including NK cells, recovered a normal profile … more propitious for fighting cancer." This result was duplicated in studies at Imperial College, London, and Ohio State University. He also cites another study involving healthy people:

> After a scant eight weeks, among those who had made a short period of meditation part of their everyday habits, significant changes had taken place in the electric activity of their brains as measured by EEG. Regions associated with positive mood and optimism (the left frontal regions) were distinctly more active compared to their earlier state or to that of the control group. And this effect reached further than the brain or the subject's mood.

According to neurologist Andrew Newberg, Director of the Center for Spirituality and the Mind at the University of Pennsylvania, meditating for as little as twelve minutes a day can

- » reduce stress, the number-one killer in America,
- » improve memory and cognition,
- » strengthen the immune system,
- » slow the aging process in the brain,
- » minimize the deterioration of diseases like Parkinson's and Alzheimer's.

Newberg and his colleagues have shown that regular meditation positively rewires the brain:

> Our brain-scan study showed that [meditation] strengthens a specific circuit—involving the prefrontal and orbital-frontal lobe, the anterior cingulated, basal ganglia, and thalamus—that would otherwise deteriorate with age. The circuit governs a wide variety of activities involved with consciousness, clarity of mind, reality formation, error detection, empathy, compassion, emotional balance and the suppression of anger and fear.

The content of the meditation doesn't matter; the act of focusing and becoming aware of your inner state is what counts. The more senses you involve the better—controlling your breathing, repeating a phrase or mantra, touching fingertips together, etc.

Initially I ignored meditation because of its association with eastern religions and New-Age mysticism. I downplayed the fact that it's been a valued discipline in Christianity from the beginning. I also suffered from the error of Naaman the leper (2 Kings 5). The prophet Elisha told this Syrian general he could be cured by dunking himself seven times in the Jordan River. Naaman rejected this as too easy but his servant finally talked him into it—and it worked!

I've done months of chemo, spent weeks preparing for and undergoing a bone marrow transplant, driven across town for radiation treatments thirty-three times but have balked at meditating for twelve minutes at home! No more. Meditation is now part of my daily regime. I've even come up with my own mantra.

Based on scores of neurological studies, Dr. Newberg recommends eight habits that improve brain health. Here are the top four from his book, *How God Changes Your Brain*:

4: Meditate

If you stay in a contemplative state for twenty minutes to an hour ... antistress hormones and neurochemicals are released throughout the body, as well as pleasure-enhancing and depression-decreasing neurotransmitters like dopamine and serotonin. Even ten to fifteen minutes of meditation appears to have significantly positive effects on cognition, relaxation, and psychological health.

3: Aerobic exercise

Exercise improves cognition and academic performance. It repairs and protects you from the neurological damage caused by stress. It enhances brain plasticity. It boosts immune function. It reduces anxiety. ... It slows down the loss of brain tissue as you age, protects you from Alzheimer's disease, and reduces your vulnerability to chronic illness.

2: Dialogue with others

If we don't exercise our language skills, large portions of the brain will not effectively interconnect with other neural structures. Dialogue requires social interaction, and the more social ties we have, the less our cognitive abilities will decline. In fact, any form of social isolation will damage important mechanisms in the brain leading to aggression, depression, and various neuropsychiatric disorders.

1: *Faith*

Faith is equivalent with hope, optimism, and the belief that
a positive future awaits us. … They [Mayo Clinic] found that
positive thinking decreases stress, helps you resist catching
the common cold, reduces your risk of coronary artery disease,
eases breathing if you have certain respiratory diseases, and
improves your coping skills during hardships. An optimistic
attitude specifically reduces the stress-eliciting cortisol levels
in your body.

"Mind-body medicine has become so widely accepted today
that it is difficult to recall when it was considered fantasy," notes
Barbara Bradley Hagerty in her book, *Fingerprints of God*:

It was not until the 1970s that scientists finally began to ac-
knowledge a connection between mind and body. … The
research flowed quickly, and showed that nonphysical things
like thoughts and emotions affect our bodies at the cellular
level just as surely as do genes or lifestyle or the medicines we
take. Emotions—particularly depression and stress—are linked
to heart attacks. They suppress the immune system as it tries
to fight the flu. One's thoughts and attitudes affect the course
of cancer and the recovery from breast cancer.

More specifically, Hagerty found out that a belief in God makes
a dramatic difference. "Turning to God rather than rejecting God
appears to boost your immune system and stave off disease nearly
five times as effectively."

My relationship with God the last few years has caused stress,
not alleviated it, which I'm sure has played a role in my ill health.
Understanding and improving that relationship are vital to getting
better.

o   o   o

"Studies have proven that people live longer
when they have an optimistic outlook."
—David Agus

HABITS OLD AND NEW

The first week in March I'm once more diagnosed with strep-pneumonia. This is getting to be an old habit. That doesn't become easier with practice. I feel as limp and washed out as a Motel 6 towel. Fortunately, I'm able to stay out of the hospital and self-medicate with three different drugs. But I can't stay out of the cancer clinic. I go back on April 11 for IVIG—intravenous immunoglobulin.

> IVIG contains the pooled, polyvalent, IgG (immunoglobulin G) extracted from the plasma of over one thousand blood donors. [Some sources say as many as ten thousand to one hundred thousand donors are needed for a complete infusion.] IVIG is given as a plasma protein replacement therapy for immune deficient patients who have decreased or abolished antibody production capabilities (http://en.wikipedia.org/wiki/Intravenous_immunoglobulin).

I don't like having the words "deficient" or "decreased capabilities" used about me but three bouts of pneumonia in seven months is nothing to cough at. I'm thankful for a little help from my friends—all ten thousand to one hundred thousand of them.

Halfway through the infusion I have a reaction. A fever and painful back spasms hit suddenly and unexpectedly. I don't remember muscle cramps on the list of possible side effects but I tend to specialize in the unusual. The symptoms subside after I'm given three different medications in quick succession.

Speaking of threes, I talked to Dr. Dax afterward and he said I was on a three-month IVIG cycle, so I have to come back twice more. I'll get pre-meds next time and hopefully avoid a repeat performance.

It was comforting to have the family over last week to remember Susie's birthday (April 12). We visited the cemetery and Nate and I cooked dinner afterward. The grandkids scampered about happily, enjoying being with four generations of a loving family with a godly heritage. Susan was such an integral part of creating both. We all miss her so much. I miss her so much.

On Friday, April 22, I think I recognize my old nemesis— pneumonia: wet cough, low energy, fever and chills. Sunday afternoon, I visit the ER with a 102-degree fever. I'm still waiting for the results of the blood tests. It could be a reaction to the IVIG infusion I got last week, or it could just be an opportunistic infection. Either way, being sick puts a kink in my schedule.

Family Traditions
Life heads in a more positive direction the last week in April. My blood work doesn't show anything unusual, so it was probably just an infection that sent me to the ER and laid me low for several days. I'm feeling better now, getting more energy daily. I should be able to handle another IVIG infusion in two weeks.

I see Dr. Cichon on Tuesday. He confirms there are no signs of carcinoma but reminds me that mine had been a fast-growing tumor, and if it was going to return it will likely do so in the eighteen months post op. Beyond that he will monitor me for five years before

I can be declared "cured." I don't like that word when it comes to cancer but I'll definitely take being "clean" for now.

Several members of my family run the BolderBOULDER 10K race with me—and 55,000 others. I haven't run that far in twenty years but I never had to walk. The course meanders through the picturesque college town and finishes in Folsom Field where the CU Buffaloes play. I enjoy the race and clocked in at seventy minutes. We might make the BolderBOULDER a family tradition.

Another tradition we've started this spring is winemaking. We call ourselves Toe Tag Winery. We have an Australian Syrah in the carboy and a Chilean Malbec in the primary fermenter (a plastic bucket). Next month we might try a chocolate raspberry port.

Winemaking is like playing with a chemistry set. The potions include percarbonates, bentonite, metabisulfate, sorbate and fining agents—yummy! The equipment isn't too expensive if amortized over several batches: hydrometer, digital thermometer, wine thief, carboys, siphons, whips and tubing of various sizes.

Directions are straightforward; chances of major explosions are slim; empty bottles are free if one has the right sort of friends. In the process, we pick up the vintner's arcane vocabulary and learn the difference between hips and shoulders, bunts and bungs, legs and lees, racking and fining.

If winemaking is an art, we are at the finger-painting stage. Practice might not make perfect but hopefully it will prove the difference between a sociable drink and salad dressing.

Jesus made as much as 180 gallons of good wine in an instant. It will take us about six months to produce thirty bottles. The first vintage from Toe Tag will be ready by Thanksgiving.

When was the last time you started a new hobby, tried a new sport, sampled a new cuisine, visited a new country, studied a new subject, bought a new toy or made a new friend?

Even nuns try on new habits once in a while.

Good Question

In June I travel to New England to spend time with friends who used to live in Colorado Springs and attended the same church Susan and I did. Then it's on to see the Farmer at His Mansion, a Christian rehabilitation center in New Hampshire. I speak at chapel while I'm there and share some of what I've been through the last four years. Afterward someone asks why I just didn't give up. Why fight so hard to stay alive?

Good question. I'm ready to go but I hang around for a few reasons:

It's not my time yet: I have things to do, people to see, books to write, grandkids to spoil, wine to make. I choose to stay engaged until my equipment fails.

I don't believe in reincarnation: I only get one outing in this theme park and I want to experience as much as I can, even if it includes rides that make me throw up.

I don't want to hurt my loved ones: I saw—and felt—the agony caused by Susan's death and I want to put off a repeat of that trauma as long as possible.

Still, life can be a heavy burden at times. Why does it have to be so stinkin' convoluted and caustic? Why does God allow all the painful iterations when he could have written a cleaner OS for creation? (Think carefully before saying he was constricted by outside forces.)

I don't have good answers for most of my "why" questions, but I choose to stick around and keep learning.

Why do you bother?

As I'm flying back from New England on Tuesday, June 28, my neighborhood is being evacuated ahead of the Waldo Canyon fire. I'm at baggage claim when my son calls from the house asking what I want him to grab. I prepared a list the day before. It was surprisingly short—photo albums, memory boxes and important papers—all things he had already loaded, along with the two carboys of Toe Tag wine, of course. Smart kid.

For more than thirty-two thousand of us in Colorado Springs, this is no drill. What would you save if you only had an hour? That's where you should be spending your time and money now.

You don't need a fire to teach you that.

o   o   o

"Each day is an opportunity to travel back into
tomorrow's past and change it."
—Robert Brault

THE HAMEL DIET

In an effort to improve my health I've hit on the novel idea of creating my own diet. While doctors and other so called experts cheat by using actual medical research to develop their programs, I've taken a more natural approach, relying solely on sixty years of eating experience and my pharmaceutically enhanced intuition.

I have settled on these ingredients so far:

- » free-range poultry from any "red" state, since it's an election year;
- » oil from olives whose virginity has been confirmed by a doctor;
- » freshly ground Ethiopian coffee beans brewed in a French press;
- » almond milk from hormone-free, grass-fed almonds;
- » whole-wheat bread baked by monks and blessed by a bishop;
- » red wine with legs good enough to star in a Vegas show;
- » any cheese that doesn't smell like it comes from between toes.

Things strictly forbidden on the Hamel Diet:

- » coffee enemas (enemas of any form should be rejected in the end);
- » any supplements sold on TV by a guy wearing a white coat;

» fish and all marine life that swim in their own pee and poop (think about it, people);

» anything fermented that you can't drink, such as sauerkraut, canned beets, sour cream;

» herbal teas that taste like grass clippings from a yard with dogs;

» tofu and any other food with the texture of congealed mucus;

» any cheese that smells like it comes from between toes.

Feel free to try the Hamel Diet for yourself. If it doesn't produce spiritual enlightenment and physical immortality, I will gladly refund your money.

Healthier Eating in Twelve Words

I've done a fair bit of reading and research on food since being diagnosed with cancer. I've gone so far as to come up with my own diet, as you've just read. However, I am not a nutritionist, dietitian, fifth-level vegan or food nazi. I don't push my views on others but I don't mind sharing what I'm learning with anyone who's interested in healthier eating.

Still reading? Let me condense dozens of books and documentaries into four foundational pads on which to build a solid diet:

Eat real food: Much of what's in stores is chemically adulterated food-like products. Look for a short list of ingredients—or none at all.

Eat whole food: Don't focus on components (such as vitamins, proteins, fats). With food, the whole is more important than the sum of its parts.

Eat fresh food: Get food in as close to its original state as possible. The fewer steps between harvesting and consuming the better.

Eat for pleasure: Food is more than fuel. Michael Pollan puts eating in perspective in his book, *In Defense of Food*:

We forget that, historically, people have eaten for a great many reasons other than biological necessity. Food is also about pleasure, about community, about family and spirituality, about our relationship to the natural world, and about expressing our identity. As long as humans have been eating meals together, eating has been as much about culture as it has been about biology.

The China Study

Of all the books on health and nutrition I've read, one of the most helpful has been *The China Study* by Dr. T. Colin Campbell. The *New York Times* has recognized the study (China-Oxford-Cornell Diet and Health Project) as the "Grand Prix of epidemiology" and the "most comprehensive large study ever undertaken of the relationship between diet and the risk of developing disease."

Based on more than four decades of research, the conclusions run counter to most popular diet books. Wikipedia lists the author's eight principles of food and health:

1. Nutrition represents the combined activities of countless food substances. The whole is greater than the sum of its parts.
2. Vitamin supplements are not a panacea for good health.
3 There are virtually no nutrients in animal-based foods that are not better provided by plants.
4. Genes do not determine disease on their own. Genes function only by being activated, or expressed, and nutrition plays a critical role in determining which genes, good and bad, are expressed.
5. Nutrition can substantially control the adverse effects of noxious chemicals.

6. The same nutrition that prevents disease in its early stages can also halt or reverse it in its later stages.

7. Nutrition that is truly beneficial for one chronic disease will support health across the board.

8. Good nutrition creates health in all areas of our existence. All parts are interconnected.

The book can be condensed in two sentences: People who eat the most animal-based foods get the most chronic disease. People who eat the most plant-based foods are the healthiest and tend to avoid chronic disease. But comedian Kathleen Madigan has a point when she says, "If God didn't mean for us to eat cows, why did he make them so easy to catch?"

Although compelling, the study is not without its flaws. Health blogger Denise Minger (http://rawfoodsos.com) has a well-reasoned critique of *The China Study* that's worth reading. She agrees with the general direction of the book but questions the science behind some of the conclusions:

> I believe the "plant-based diet doctors" got a lot of things right, and a diet of whole, unprocessed plant foods (i.e., Real Food) can bring tremendous health improvements for people who were formerly eating a low-nutrient, high-crap diet. Especially short term. But I also believe this type of diet achieves some of its success by accident, and that the perks of eliminating processed junk are inaccurately attributed to eliminating all animal foods. So the goal of this critique is to shed light on the areas where the "plant-based science" is a little, um, wilted.

Minger contends the authors oversimplify the evidence and that their conclusions are too sweeping. Like Homer Simpson says,

"You could use facts to prove anything that's even remotely true."
    My conclusions: Vegetarians and vegans have their own issues.
Animal products may not all be anathema.
    All things in moderation.
    Enjoy.

o   o   o

"No people on earth worry more about the health consequences
    of their food choices than we Americans do—
and no people suffer from as many diet-related problems."
    —Michael Pollan

SYPTOM FREE, NOT PAIN FREE

D r. Cichon gave me a clean bill of health today (November 27). It's been fourteen months since he cut a tumor out of my face and just over a year since my last radiation and chemo treatments. (He takes no responsibility for the brain damage, since that's self-inflicted.) Eighty percent of the time a squamous cell carcinoma returns, it's within the first year. The next six months are also critical and the odds of a relapse continue to decline until the five-year mark when I would be considered "cured."

I don't like that word. Symptom free—for now—is more realistic.

As to my original lymphoma, which I've had twice, I get my next CT scan in a few weeks. It will probe for cancerous growth from skull to knees. "Normal" would be a nice word to hear afterward. I will also have the results sent to Dr. Leppard to see what's wrong with my left shoulder. It's not improving with rest but getting worse. She will no doubt order an MRI to figure out the cause and the best treatment option. I don't like the pain and limitations this problem imposes and want to get back to more strenuous exercise.

We are indeed "fearfully and wonderfully made," but our equipment wears out and maintenance becomes more challenging with age.

And expensive.

I finally got the bill for my radiation treatments last year. Thirty-three treatments over three months cost $107,437. Add this to the $180,000 for two years of Rituxan, plus the price of seventeen other chemo sessions, seven surgeries, multiple hospital stays, a bone marrow transplant and a car accident and the retail price of my medical care the last four years has climbed into the seven figures. Who knows how much the insurance companies actually paid?

To put that number in perspective, the cost of keeping me alive is approaching the price tag of a single Tomahawk missile—$1,410,000. Yes, the Tomahawk is faster and more lethal than me but it can only be used once whereas I've been in service for sixty years. And I'm a better listener.

Repeat Offender

I'm ending 2012 the way I began it—with pneumonia. Having had it five times now I've become more proactive in treating it. As a repeat offender I've been on different antibiotics. This time I'm trying cefuroxime, a second-generation cephalosporin antibiotic.

I'm thankful for these wonder drugs but they come at a price. I didn't realize until recently that almost all antibiotics (bacteria that kill other bacteria) have been developed from a single source, an order of microorganisms called Actinomycetales. As we put these bacteria in everything from medicine to food to soap, other bacteria evolve ways to resist them. At some point the scale will tip against us. In some areas it already has. Dr. Eben Alexander reports a recent example:

> In 1996, doctors discovered a new bacterial strain harboring DNA for a gene coding for *Klebiella pneumonia carbapenemase*, or KPC, an enzyme that conferred antibiotic resistance on its host bacterium. … The strain immediately got the attention of doctors all over the world when it was discovered that KPC

could potentially render a bacteria that absorbed it resistant not just to some current antibiotics, but to all of them. If a toxic antibiotic-proof strain of bacteria (one whose nontoxic cousin is ubiquitous in our bodies) got loose in the general population, it would have a field day with the human race.

This is one reason to avoid hospitals when you can. Every year more than two million people get drug-resistant bacterial infections there, and more than ninety-nine thousand patients die from preventable causes.

My last few CT scans have shown scarring in my lungs, which makes me more vulnerable to infection. I never had pneumonia before my bone marrow transplant so there must also be a specific hole in my rebuilt immune system, a tolerable nuisance for still being alive.

Despite being reminded every few months, I forget (thankfully) the wallop pneumonia packs. It's like being tackled by an All-Pro linebacker while keeled over with the flu. The days are long, the nights achingly longer. At least I get to spend them at home.

Based on my track record, I can expect return bouts in 2013. Next time I might try medical marijuana. It would be among the mildest of the few dozen drugs I've taken in recent years. I've been on prescriptions that have killed the rich and famous. I've had derivatives of mustard gas and liquid platinum repeatedly injected into me by nurses in masks and protective gear. What's a little Delta-9-Tetrahydrocannabinol (THC)?

My lungs aren't the only things giving me problems. My left shoulder has been bothering me for months. Physical therapy and rest haven't helped so I finally get an MRI that reveals a torn rotator cuff and other complications. Time to revisit the surgeon who repaired my right shoulder (twice) to learn what my options are. (Another surgery as it turns out.)

I know professional writers are prone to self-inflicted liver damage but no one warned me about possible joint injuries brought on by a lifetime of typing. Or it could just be that I'm getting older.

Painful Nonsense

No pain, no gain.

Nonsense.

What's painful is gainful only part of the time. While pain serves a vital role in keeping us alive, it can also be grossly overbearing, notoriously unreliable and sadistically redundant. "I'm not saying the body isn't amazing in many ways, " admits A. J. Jacobs in *Drop Dead Healthy*:

> But at the same time, the body has many deeply embedded bugs. ... And pain is one of the crudest, most primal systems. Pain is so unsubtle. Couldn't evolution (or God) have found a better way to alert us that we stubbed our toe rather than this sensation that makes us curse the day our mom and dad met at the college cafeteria?
>
> Pain can erupt with no cause, linger for years, even appear in a phantom limb. And here's one of pains most sadistic qualities: If you suffer from chronic pain (as 70 million Americans do), it often doesn't ebb as the body heals. It often gets worse. Pain begets pain. The neural pathways become smoother, the message stronger.

I write this on the eve of my third rotator cuff surgery—and I only have two shoulders! It will no doubt be followed by a slow and painful recovery. I just wanted to post this paltry protest against pain before the oxycontin kicks in.

○   ○   ○

"Who still thinks there is some device (if only he could find it),
which will make pain not to be pain. It doesn't really matter
whether you grip the arms of the dentist's chair
or let your hands lie in your lap.
The drill goes on."
—C. S. Lewis

VALENTINE'S DAY

My daughter Julie is my date for Valentine's Day. She takes me to a romantic medical center where I have my eighth surgery in the last five years. It's my third rotator cuff surgery. Once again the procedure goes well. True to form, the days following have been terrible. Pain, fatigue and an allergic reaction combine to make me one sick puppy.

This time around I try various forms of medical marijuana to dull the screaming echoes of the operation. This herb has been widely used since caveman days with great success but my doctor's malpractice insurance won't let him prescribe it. (Don't want docs dispensing dangerous drugs now, do we?) I have high (sic) hopes but get lousy results. It makes me dizzy and nauseated. And disappointed, because I wanted a more natural way to mitigate the pain.

Take it from a drug tramp; abstinence is the best policy—except for caffeine, which is a vitamin not a drug. When you have to use, choose the poison with the smallest metabolic footprint.

Whatever was going on with my lungs beforehand hasn't cleared up and my immune system is busy fighting off something. I have no energy and the lack of drive reminds me of how I felt during the worst of the chemo.

Time isn't helping the situation. Four weeks out from surgery and I'm still losing weight and energy. I almost fainted in the grocery checkout line yesterday. The lady behind me prayed for me and bought me a bottle of water. Very nice. I found myself crying on the way out of the store because of the weakness.

I'm back in a sling, which makes mundane movements a challenge. Try taping one arm to your side and doing these everyday tasks with the other hand:

» uncorking a wine bottle
» shoveling snow
» blowing your nose
» peeling a banana
» tying your shoes
» flossing
» cleaning your glasses
» opening a jar of olives
» putting on socks
» buttering toast
» answering emails
» hooking a bra (just guessing here)

Where can you find workarounds for these challenges? A secondhand store, of course.

Spring Slump

Fatigue continues to be my nemesis. I haven't been this flat since my bone marrow transplant. Sleep is sketchy, energy is limited and margins are gone. Six weeks post-op and I still need pain pills to get through the day and a sleeping pill to get through the night. When I sit, it's like being velcroed to the chair. It could just be the cumulative effect of five years of unremitting medical drama and attendant emotional trauma. Alfred Hitchcock once said, "What is drama, after all, but life with the dull bits cut out." I could do with a less-dramatic lifestyle.

More doctors and tests in the never-ending search to discover what's wrong with me (below the neck). I'm having everything checked from possible allergies to immunoglobulin levels. So far all my scans and lab work haven't revealed anything too far from the norm. It hasn't helped that I fell in the street playing kickball with the grandkids on Father's Day and separated my shoulder. Yes, the one I had repaired a few months back.

The physical is hard enough without being made more difficult by the absence of spiritual solace. I used to believe everything happens for a reason and that God's presence would see us through anything. This may be true but it hasn't been my experience the last few years. I can assume God is sustaining me since I'm still here, but that's not much consolation when I want someone to lean on and bear me up.

The dissonance between what I believe and what I feel is discouraging. If it lies solely in my power to fix it, I don't know how.

Moving On

After fifteen years in the same place—a record—I sold my house and much of what's in it to reduce expenses and simplify my lifestyle. This way I'll be able to afford my habits awhile longer: buying prescription meds, writing books, making wine, spending time with interesting people and searching for truth.

There are seasons during which we need stuff and space, such as when we're building a career or raising a family. And there are times later in life to shed and simplify rather than filling up basements, garages and storage units with artifacts. I applied the One-Year Rule in paring down my possessions: If I haven't touched it in a year I probably don't need it.

Downsizing can be hard if we equate wealth with the amount of stuff we own or space we control. But to me it's liberating because I think of wealth in terms of freedom, flexibility and the ability to focus.

I almost forgot the fourth "F."

Fun.

○   ○   ○

"Taking it with you isn't nearly so important
as making it last until you're ready to go."
—Author Unknown

FAUSTIAN BARGAIN

Anything that begins with "hypo-" and ends with "-nemia" can't be good, but at least I now know what I have. In the summer of 2013 I finally learn the probable cause of my poor health—hypogammaglobulinemia:

> A disorder caused by a lack of B-lymphocytes and a resulting low level of immunglobulins (antibodies) in the blood. Immunoglobulins play a dual role in the immune response by recognizing foreign antigens and triggering a biological response that eliminates the antigen. Antibody deficiency is associated with recurrent infections.

My immune system no longer makes enough antibodies to fight off certain attackers like pneumococcus, which explains my frequent bouts of pneumonia, susceptibility to infections and lack of energy.

One of the ironies of modern oncology is that almost everything given to fight cancer is carcinogenic. In my case the treatment for lymphoma has punched a gaping hole in my immune system. A retrospective study from Memorial Sloan-Kettering Cancer Center found that thirty-nine percent of patients with B-cell lymphoma like mine who got the drug rituximab also got hypogammaglobulinemia.

The risk is greater in patients who received maintenance rituximab.

Previously in this book I've written in glowing terms about rituximab, aka Rituxan, of which I've had more than thirty doses. Despite the good press, this ungrateful wonder drug has turned around and bitten me in the immune system!

There's no cure for hypogammaglobulinemia and I'll have to get painful and expensive infusions of IVIG (intravenous immunoglobulin) every four weeks for the rest of my life. I had a bad reaction to an IVIG infusion last year that landed me in the ER, so we'll have to figure out a better way to deliver the goods.

Chemo is a Faustian bargain but one I would make again since it's kept me around long enough to finish this book.

And to start on the sequel.

o   o   o

"I'll take a medication when I need it when the time comes,
if the benefits clearly outweigh the risks.
But I won't expect to get something for nothing."
—Katrina Firkin

EPILOGUE

I've been smitten by physical and spiritual infirmities during the past five years, smothered by fatigue and pain most of that time, and supported by family and friends throughout. The latter are the reason for fighting through the former. But are there good reasons for sharing my troubles with others? Everybody has problems; why draw attention to mine? Why not suffer in silence or shrink away from people so as not to be a burden?

I have my reasons:

Misery loves company: So does happiness for that matter, and every state in between. It's human nature to need community. Loneliness makes everything worse. Isolation kills.

I'm a writer: "Why do we do it, we writers?" Philip Yancey asks. "I think we do it because each of us has nothing else to offer but a living point of view that differentiates us from every other person on the planet. We must tell our stories to someone." It's in my nature to analyze, annotate and annunciate my experiences. I've also been known to alliterate on occasion.

I have a third reason but refuse to give it because lists with three points smack of sermons.

Life as Paraprosdokian

A paraprosdokian is a figure of speech in which the latter part of a sentence or phrase is surprising or unexpected and frequently humorous. It's a prissy word for one-liners and it works on the same principle of misdirection as a joke. It's a proverb with a punch line, an axiom with an attitude. Here are a few of my favorites:

» The last thing I want to do is hurt you—but it's still on my list.
» I may have my faults—but being wrong isn't one of them.
» The early bird gets the worm—but the second mouse gets the cheese.
» My play was a complete success—the audience was a failure.
» I didn't say it was your fault—I said I was blaming you.
» A bird in the hand—is going to poop in it.

Life resembles a paraprosdokian when the latter part takes a surprising or unexpected turn. Sometimes the change is cruel and ironic rather than humorous. In my case:

» I never went to college—but my only debt as I enter my sixties is for my children's student loans.
» I spend decades in Bible study and ministry—and wind up with debilitating questions and doubt.
» I survive three bouts of cancer, a bone marrow transplant and a serious car accident—and my wife dies two weeks after I finish treatment.

Despite these bruised and painful elbows, life isn't all bent. I have much to be thankful for, including a great family, close friends and the chance to pursue my passions. And who knows what other fun plot twists the final chapters might contain?

For my part, I'm trying hard to make mine a story worth retelling—and not just a cautionary tale.

o   o   o

"Life is a great big canvas,
and you should throw all the paint on it you can."
—Danny Kaye

ACKNOWLEDGMENTS

I wouldn't be here today without these people—and wouldn't want to be.

My family who has shown practical love daily:
Susan first and foremost, Aaron and Sarah, Nate and Jenn, Julie and Alan, Matt and Michelle, Mom and Dad, Linda and Sarah, Ruth and Andrew, Tom, Bruce and Janet, Aaron and Karen, Kathy and Herb, Katie and Pat, Martin, Laura and my extended family.

The guys I meet with regularly who have been empathetic and encouraging:
Brethren Happy Hour: Bob Larson and Kim Carlson. Old Chicago Literary Society: Craig Glass and Ron Lee. Lunch Bunch: Al Butkus and Don Hoeckle.

My mates at the office (Agia Sophia):
Dave Rickert, Harriet Lee, Amelia and Constantin Prajescu, Matt and Kristin Kennedy, Father Anthony and Elizabeth Karbo.

The Professionals:
Doctors: Dax Kurbegov, Mark Brunvand, Larry Dillon, David

Weinstein, John Cichon, Mark Hazuka, Bruce Suckling, Robert Hoyer and Robert Nathan.

Nurses: Brenda Hicks, Sharon Britain and the wonderful staff at Memorial Cancer Center. Anne Emmons, Michelle Ford and the caring crew at Memorial Infusion Center.

Physical Therapists: Dave Conlin, Mike Buckler and Kelly Haddock.

Attorneys: Jeff Rowes and Robert Anderson.

Organizations:
Leukemia & Lymphoma Society, www.leukemia-lymphoma.org.
Institute for Justice, www.ij.org.
More Marrow Donors, www.moremarrowdonors.org.

And to the hundreds of others who have prayed for me and encouraged me along the way. I owe you all a debt of gratitude I can never repay.

ABOUT THE AUTHOR

MIKE HAMEL has written many books including a trilogy dealing with faith in the marketplace. His fiction includes the eight-volume juvenile fiction series Matterhorn the Brave (www.MatterhorntheBrave.com), the TLC series for young readers (www.TLCStories.com) and the illustrated *Lizzy the Leatherback*.

Prior to becoming a full-time writer in 1996, Mike served as a teaching pastor for fifteen years and helped plant two churches. He also served as a resource director and editor at Interest Ministries in Wheaton, Illinois.

Mike lives in Colorado Springs and blogs at OPEN Mike, www://mikehamel.word-press.com.

www.ingramcontent.com/pod-product-compliance
Lightning Source LLC
Chambersburg PA
CBHW061349280526
45784CB00001B/190